CONTENTS

SCIENTIFIC FEATURES OF MODERN MEDICINE

I

A SKETCH OF THE NORMAL HUMAN BODY

In his profound book, "Of the Proficience and Advancement of Learning," Francis Bacon, writing at the beginning of the seventeenth century, speaks of medicine as follows: "Medicine is a science which hath been . . . more professed than laboured, and yet more laboured than advanced; the labour having been, in my judgement, rather in circle than in progression. For I find much iteration, but small addition." At that moment the world was standing at the threshold of a great medical advance. The circle of medievalism had already been broken by the anatomist Vesalius and his contemporaries; the physiologist Harvey was soon to announce the discovery of the circulation of the blood; and the labors of men of medicine were thereafter to result in progression. During the seventeenth and eighteenth centuries progression was destined to be slow; during the nineteenth it took on a sudden and unexampled acceleration. Three hundred years have now elapsed since Bacon wrote, and the progress has never been so swift as it is to-day. Each twelvemonth ends with a record of great achievements, and each new year begins with a clearer vision forward. Notwithstanding this we frequently meet with a distrust of the efficiency of medicine, a feeling that the physician knows far too little concerning disease and its cure, and a tendency to turn toward strange cults, making fair promises. Such distrust is as old as medicine itself. Its cause is complex, and I shall not now try to analyze it.[1] I do not believe that it is justified. Doubting is indeed an entirely legitimate form of mental exercise. The man of science who is not a doubter has no claim to honorable standing. He who doubts not is dead to science. But not all doubts are equally estimable. There are those that betray much knowledge and those that betray little. Goethe and Browning did not contradict one another, although the one wrote, "Doubt grows with knowledge," and the other, "Who knows most, doubts not."

Whatever distrust of medical potency may now exist, arises largely from ignorance of the human body and the present status of medical science. Among many persons this ignorance is extraordinarily great. It is strange to find thinking, reasoning, feeling men and women, who were born with their bodies, who have lived long lives and grown old with their bodies, who have clung to them in sickness and in health, for better, for worse, who have used them for every variety of human service, and yet deliberately hold themselves aloof from a knowledge of bodily affairs. I suspect that we have here an inheritance, through many generations, of the medieval notion of the vileness of the body, a notion which is out of keeping with the enlightened science of to-day. This science shows within ourselves wondrous mechanisms and adaptations, which ought to arouse a man's admiration if he possesses a truly esthetic sense. The medical profession is occasionally criticized for its alleged failure to take the laity into its confidence and to serve as teachers as well as practitioners of its principles. I shall not here discuss the question

---

[1] For a fuller discussion of this distrust, see p. 165.

in how far a physician is morally bound to be a pedagogue. But in accepting the Jesup Lectureship, I was influenced largely by the thought that through it I might perhaps be of service to both the medical profession and an intelligent public by telling the public something of what medical leaders are doing.

A recent writer has drawn a graphic picture of the three stages that appear in the history of medicine — those of dogma, of empiricism, and of modern science. Dogma was rife until the close of the Middle Ages; empiricism characterized the Renaissance and the centuries immediately following; while modern science is a matter of decades. However sharply differentiated are these stages, something of science characterized the earlier ones, while something of both dogma and empiricism, though forever dethroned, still persists. It would be fatuous to disparage the inheritance with which medicine entered upon its present stage, but one would be blind not to recognize its truly wonderful growth under the influence of the scientific spirit of our generation. The stimulus to this growth came partly from many extraneous and now familiar sources. The discovery of oxygen, the establishment of the theory of the conservation of energy, the overthrow of the mystical doctrine of vital force, the discovery of protoplasm, the promulgation of the cell theory of organic structure, and the formulation of the theory of evolution — all contributed their share. The chief agents through which the great change has come are the laboratory, now little more than threescore and ten years old, and the method of orderly experimentation which the laboratory alone could foster.

One of the first and most essential steps in the modern expansion was the acquisition of a better understanding of the human body in its normal condition of health. Here much has been accomplished. Though human anatomy is still far from being a completed science, the gross structure of the body was appreciated early. When we submit the body to a physical examination, externally and internally, we find it to consist, first, of a number of easily recognized parts, which have long been known as organs. The existence of most of the organs of the human body were recognized before the Christian era. This knowledge was at first gained doubtless chiefly from observation of the bodies of men killed in battle. It was not until the famous school of Alexandria had reached the zenith of its glory in the third century before Christ that the human body became actually dissected for purposes of study. Later, dissection fell into ill repute, and it has required modern science to free it finally from obloquy and prejudice. If we proceed farther in our physical examination and look carefully at any one of the various organs, we find it to be composed of a small number of materials, varying in appearance and easily recognizable by the naked eye. To these materials the name tissues has been given, and we may distinguish such as muscular tissue, nervous tissue, connective tissue, epithelial tissue, bony tissue, fatty and cartilaginous tissue. Though the existence of tissues is plainly obvious to an observer, it was not until one hundred years ago that their structural significance was clearly recognized — first, by a French anatomist, Bichat, who classified them and pointed out their distribution within the body. It is easy now, in the days of powerful microscopes and intricate microscopical methods, to carry the physical examination of organs and tissues into the realm of what was undreamed of by the ancients, and the significance of which has been appreciated only within the lifetime of still living men. But Bichat did not realize that all tissues are com-

posed of recognizable particles, now called cells, of living substance, now called protoplasm. Moreover, cytologists do not stop here, but differentiate, within the cell, nucleus and cytoplasm, centrosome and chromosomes; the ultra-microscope is leading us on toward a sight of still smaller components; theories of the physical structure of protoplasm are hotly discussed; and interchangeable states of solution and gelation are thought to occur within it.

Living substance, in itself soft and delicate and gelatinous, is permeated throughout by non-living water and by non-living solids, which are antecedents or products of cell activities. Having said this, I ought to confess that often it is a practical impossibility to decide what within a cell is living and what is not living. Moreover, when we attempt to submit the living substance and its contents to chemical analysis, our first step results in its death and chemical change, and we have no longer living, but only dead, substance in our test-tubes. We are thus at first baffled in our endeavor to determine the actual chemical structure of protoplasm, and indeed we are here still in the realm of hypothesis. But we are, nevertheless, making progress in learning the bricks or chemical cleavage products, which result from the demoli-tion of protoplasm and of which it is built up. All the various chemical substances are composed of comparatively few of the chemical elements. Only carbon, hydrogen, oxygen, nitrogen, sulphur, phosphorus, chlorine, sodium, potassium, calcium, magnesium, iodine, silicon, fluorine, manganese, and iron are known to occur in every human body. But these are capable of entering into a long series of permutations and combinations with one another, the various organic com-pounds rarely possessing the simplicity of composition that occurs in inorganic nature. Thus we find many representatives of the ever interesting group of proteins, huge molecules containing hundreds, or even thousands, of atoms, which seem to be arranged in most intricate patterns. For no protein has this pattern yet been fully made out, but it is believed that many of the atoms are grouped into the so-called amino-acids, and that the protein molecules represent still more intricate groupings of these groups, in themselves complex. Besides a considerable number of proteins there occur in protoplasm starches and sugars and fats of various kinds and compositions, water, and various salts. The salts probably exist, in part at least, as ions, electrically charged atoms or groups of atoms, which are chemically combined with the proteins, thus adding to the latter's complexity.

The scientific physician must understand not only the morphological and chemical structure of the bodily machine, but the way in which it acts. However complex structure appears to be, it is simple when compared with function. The modern physiologist looks upon the body as a machine, a machine in which physical and chemical processes are constantly occurring in orderly sequence and in which energy, no more created here than elsewhere, is being constantly changed from one form to another. Function is thus the expression of physical and chemical principles, and it is the physiologist's endeavor to resolve the vital phenomena of organs, tissues, and cells into their physical and chemical components. He has already gone a long way in doing this; but, as might be expected of the science of the life process, every problem solved leaves other problems awaiting solution, and with every mystery mastered still other mysteries lure and baffle.

Let me enumerate some of the chief functions of the body. The heart by the force of its beats, which are contractions of its muscular walls, moves the blood, receiving it from the veins and propelling it along the arteries. The actions of the heart's valves, the sequence of activity and the dynamic relations of its parts, and its regulation by the nervous system are fairly well understood. We can point with reasonable certainty to the spot at which the beat originates, but we are not agreed as to the nature of the stimulus which sets it off four thousand times during each hour of our lives, or whether the stimulus acts primarily on nervous or muscular tissue.

The lungs serve to introduce oxygen into, and to remove carbonic acid from, the blood. For this purpose the lungs and chest act together like a bellows, the moving power residing in the muscles of the walls and floor of the chest, which are under the control of the nervous system. We understand much of the pneumatic conditions and the nervous relations of the process, but we are still trying to learn in what manner the exchange of oxygen and carbonic acid between the air and the blood occurs.

The successive steps in the digestion of food occurring in the stomach and intestine are recognized in the main.

From earliest times the liver has been misunderstood, often maligned, and always the subject of hypothesis. The physiology of to-day recognizes in it a considerable number of important functions. Like certain parts of a plant's body, its cells serve as a storehouse for such of the body's starch as is not needed for immediate use, and on the demand of the tissues they give this out to the blood in the form of easily transported sugar. The liver is, in fact, the body's "sugar trust" — without, however, employing the peculiar methods that have made famous its modern namesake. It manufactures and give to the intestine bile, which is an important aid to the digestion and absorption of fats, and an important

medium for the removal of certain waste products of the
tissues' activities. It manufactures and gives to the kidneys
urea, another waste product, whose prompt removal from
the body is essential to health. To some extent the liver is
capable of protecting the body by rendering inert a variety of
poisonous substances, such as those that may have been produced within the intestine in the course of digestion, those
that may have been caused by disease germs, and even such
poisons as strychnine, morphine, and metallic salts, which
may have been taken by the individual with good or evil
intent. Various as are the known activities of the liver, it
is probable that future research will reveal still others of
great importance.

The pancreas manufactures and sends to the intestine a
liquid which contains three ferments capable of digesting
proteins, fats, and starches, respectively. The kidneys and
their connected organs remove from the body a variety of
chemical substances, both organic and inorganic, which are
the end products of the body's chemical changes, and the
retention of which would be harmful.

Glands are an endless source of interest. We know that
from them appear characteristic liquids; but why, from the
uniform store of materials in the blood supplied to all glands
in common, the salivary glands secrete saliva, the glands of
the stomach gastric juice, the liver bile, and the kidneys
urine, and as to what physical principles are involved in the
passage of the widely different components of these various
juices through the gland cells, we are much in doubt. Within
only a few years we have learned that besides producing and
excreting through their ducts their characteristic juices,
glands give back to the blood equally characteristic substances, many of which are indispensable to the continued

activity of other organs and to life itself. This process has come to be known as internal secretion, and the same term is applied to the substances thus produced. Thus the liver gives to the blood sugar and urea. The pancreas gives to the blood, apparently only through the activity of certain peculiar groups of its cells, a substance which, in some way still to be determined, plays an important rôle in the chemical changes undergone by sugar within the body. Removal or serious disease of the pancreas results in the accumulation of sugar in the blood and its constant loss from the body in the urine, which are the striking symptoms of diabetes. An internal secretion of unknown nature seems to come from the kidney. The peculiar bodies called the thyroids appear to produce a substance which is of great importance to certain nutritive activities of the brain. The absence of this substance may lead in the young to the peculiar form of idiocy called cretinism, and in the adult to a disease known as myxedema, both of which are characterized by symptoms of mental deterioration. An excess of thyroid secretion, on the other hand, may lead to an equally distressing disease, known as exophthalmic goiter. Still other organs yield equally striking internal secretions. In fact, internal secretions seem to constitute one of the chief media by which parts of the body act upon other parts, often in the most profound and unexpected ways. The principle of such coöperation in bodily activity has been discovered only recently, and we are quite prepared to learn at any time of new instances of it.

One of the most active fields of research in physiology to-day is that which deals with the chemical changes undergone by the body in the process of living. Half a century ago this was largely a matter of speculation. Now we recognize that, with its living and its non-living substances inextricably intermingled, the body constitutes an intensive chemical laboratory in which there is ever occurring a vast congeries of chemical reactions; both constructive and destructive processes go on; new protoplasm takes the place of old. We can analyze the income of the body and we can analyze its output, and from these data we can learn much concerning the body's chemistry. A great improvement in the method of such work has recently been secured by the device of inclosing the person who is the subject of the experiment in a respiration calorimeter. This is an air-tight chamber, artificially supplied with a constant stream of pure air, and from which the expired air, laden with the products of respiration, is withdrawn for purposes of analysis. The subject may remain in the chamber for days, the composition of all food and all excreta being determined, and all heat that is given off being measured. Favorable conditions are thus established for an exact study of many problems of nutrition. The difficulties increase when we attempt to trace the successive steps in the corporeal pathway of molecule and atom. Yet these secrets of the vital process are also gradually being revealed. When we remember that it is in this very field of nutrition that there exist great popular ignorance and a special proneness to fad and prejudice, we realize how practically helpful are such exact studies of metabolism.

I have likened the body to a machine. A more fitting simile would be that of an intricate industrial plant, in which varied machines work to produce a certain output. The first essential in such an establishment is order. The work of each machine must be methodical; its raw material must be supplied in just the right quantity and at just the right time;

its products, both useful products and wastes, must be removed promptly and taken to their destinations; and a harmonious adjustment of the labors of the respective parts of the plant must be continually maintained, if confusion and chaos are not to reign. The human body possesses two mechanisms for the maintenance of order and harmony among its varied parts, — the blood circulating through heart, arteries, capillaries, and veins, and conveying material substances, and the nervous system conveying immaterial nervous impulses. Nothing illustrates so well the relations of bodily functions as a consideration of these two systems.

The blood consists of a liquid part, the plasma, and a large number of minute, floating cells, or cell-like particles, called corpuscles. The plasma is capable of holding in solution a great variety of solid substances. It is the medium by which food and drink and drugs are conveyed to all portions of the organism, carbonic acid to the lungs, and other wastes to the excretory glands. Products of protoplasmic action which are the result of internal secretion and are to be used elsewhere than in their place of origin, are shipped by way of the plasma to their destinations. Those toxic products of excessive activity that are known as fatigue substances are transported by the plasma to all tissues, and thus make it possible that the fatigue of a working organ may be extended even to those that have been resting. Whatever a tissue requires it receives from the store available in the blood plasma, and whatever it is to give up passes to the same medium.

The blood corpuscles are of three kinds — blood plates, red corpuscles or erythrocytes, and white corpuscles or leucocytes. The blood plates are a comparatively recent discovery, and their functions are not yet well understood.   The very abundant erythrocytes have long been known for their power of absorbing large quantities of oxygen, and in the course of evolution they seem to have become differentiated for the express duty of conveying to the tissues this essential gas. That this power is adapted to the bodily needs is shown by the fact that life in high altitudes, where the actual oxygen content of the air is relatively low, leads to a marked increase in the number of erythrocytes, and thus to an increased power on the part of the blood of absorbing oxygen.   Until recent years the leucocytes have been regarded as humble and insignificant members of the organic colony, but they have now risen to a dignity that is surpassed by few other cells.   Like the amœba they possess the power of independent motion, and like nomads they wander at will.   I say "at will" fancifully.   We have no reason to believe that leucocytes possess consciousness.   When it pleases them they allow themselves to be carried along in the blood stream, but ever and anon they forsake the blood-vessels, push their way through the walls, and roam up and down among the tissues.   It is possible that they act as carriers of food, such as fats and proteins, when these substances are ready to enter the tissues after the digestive ferments have dealt with them.   They assist in the peculiar and often life-saving process of coagulating blood.   They seem to be factors in maintaining the desired chemical composition of the blood plasma.   They probably manufacture substances that are destructive to bacteria.   And, lastly, they engulf worn-out body substance, living bacteria, and other matter foreign to the body, should such be present, and thus protect the body from harmful agencies.[1]

[1] See also pp. 45, 77 and 79.

Pumped by the heart, the blood circulates in arteries, capillaries, and veins throughout the body to its remotest parts and back again to the heart.   In the thin-walled capillaries its liquid plasma exudes into the interstitial spaces of the tissues, accompanied by numbers of leucocytes, and the two together constitute the lymph.   It is only through the lymph that the exchange between blood and tissue is effected.

Even with the elaborate blood system with its many functions the diversified body without other agency would still be unable to live a unified life.   To harmonize, correlate, and unify is the special function of the nervous system.   Without a nervous system our members might exhibit a certain degree of spontaneity, but it would be the spontaneity of unbridled license, and anarchy would soon put an end to us. For more than two thousand years men have been endeavoring to fathom the mysteries of brain and nerve, and their ultimate problems seem now as enigmatical as ever.   Even a rational idea of the structural basis of nervous action has been acquired only within three decades, and there are some biologists who are still skeptical of this.   According to the prevalent conception, the nerve-cell, now called neurone, is the unit of nervous structure.   Like other cells, it possesses a central, nucleated body of microscopic size, but unlike other cells, there extend far outward from its body in various directions delicate filaments.   The numerous, comparatively short, and much-branched filaments are called dendrites; the few, comparatively long and little-branched, axones.   A human nervous system, with its brain, spinal cord, ganglia, and nerves, is a mass of neurones.   The bodies of the neurones and their dendrites lie mostly within the brain, spinal cord, and ganglia, in more or less definitely localized masses.

The axones are mostly collected together into definite bundles or tracts, of which some lie within the brain and spinal cord, but many extend outward and, as the constituent nerve-fibers of nerves, reach all parts of the body. Through the nerves all organs and tissues are in communication with the brain or spinal cord, and only through the brain or spinal cord do organs and tissues possess the possibility of communicating with one another. Neurones, while often in contiguity and seemingly inextricably mingled, do not appear to be actually continuous with one another. Their number is legion, and through them the infinitely complex work of the nervous system is performed in an orderly, methodical manner. The messages which they transmit are called by the physiologist nervous impulses. Many theories of the nature of nervous impulses have been proposed, and though no theory is wholly satisfactory, we believe that in them certain physical, probably electrical, and chemical processes are involved. Each nerve-fiber seems to conduct impulses in one direction only. Outside the brain or spinal cord certain of the fibers conduct only from the tissues and toward the central nervous system, while certain others only in the opposite direction. Every organ seems to possess both of these afferent, or centripetal, and efferent, or centrifugal, fibers, and thus is able both to send and to receive impulses. Incoming impulses inform the brain or cord of the physiological state of the particular organ from which they come; they may give rise to sensations, and are then called sensory. The most striking functions of purely sensory nerves are those of the so-called special senses. Outgoing impulses are never in themselves sensory, although the brain actions that inaugurate many of them may be accompanied by conscious acts of the will. They inform the organs or tissues what to do under the circumstances. The following is a classification of the known varieties of nerve-fibers, according to their functions.

Afferent
- Excitatory
  - Sensory: controlling sensations of sight, hearing, smell, taste, pressure, temperature, pain, etc.
  - Reflex: inducing reflex actions through efferent fibers.
- Inhibitory: inhibiting reflex actions.

Efferent
- Excitatory
  - Motor: supplying voluntary muscles, the heart, and the muscles of arteries, stomach, intestines, etc.
  - Secretory: supplying salivary glands, glands of the stomach, and the pancreas, sweat-glands, etc.
- Inhibitory: inhibiting the activities of the muscles and glands.

Within the brain and spinal cord the various nerve-fibers, grouped into different bundles, offer definite routes for the conduction of nervous impulses. In some the impulses pass upward, in others downward, in still others from side to side. Through them the organs and tissues communicate with the various parts of the brain and spinal cord, and these in turn communicate with one another.

A single act, however simple it may appear to be, usually involves many nervous phenomena. Thus the voluntary contraction of one's biceps muscle means the transmission, not only of excitatory impulses to the biceps itself, but of inhibitory impulses to its antagonist, the triceps; other excitatory and inhibitory impulses to adjacent muscles for the purpose of inducing in them just the right degree of tension in order that the biceps may be aided; dilating impulses to the arteries of the various contracting muscles and constricting impulses to arteries elsewhere, in order to supply the muscles with more blood; impulses to the heart to beat more strongly, in order that the demands of the arteries for blood may be met; increased motor impulses to the muscles of respiration; increased secretory impulses to the sweat-glands and dilating impulses to their arteries; and perhaps other nervous impulses to other organs. If, moreover, we realize that with each one of these separate actions special afferent nervous impulses go to the nervous system announcing the nature and extent of the action, we may in our bewilderment well wonder why a mere innocent contraction of the biceps does not bring in its train an attack of nervous prostration. Gay critics of the medical profession, anti-this, and anti-that, who wonder why the problems of health and disease have not been solved long ago, have little conception of the intricacies of the human body.

One of the greatest achievements of the modern physiology of the nervous system has been the exploration of the various parts of the brain and spinal cord and the discovery that each part has its own specific work to do. The parts that are composed chiefly of the bodies of nerve-cells are known as nerve-centers, and it is customary to picture the brain and cord as consisting largely of innumerable centers connected with one another by tracts of nerve-fibers. Along the whole length of the cord there is a series of such functional centers, which deal with the activities of the muscles of the trunk and limbs and some of the abdominal organs. The bulb, or medulla oblongata, is a mass of most important centers dealing with such essential features as breathing and the actions of the heart, the arteries, and the glands. In the much-folded outer layer, or cortex, of the cerebrum lie the innumerable centers whose activities are accompanied by consciousness, and here we locate the volitional factors of locomotion, the movements of arms, hands and fingers, speech, sight, hearing, taste, smell, and touch.   Here also are mediated the psychic processes of perception, conscious memory, the association of ideas, and the thousand and one features of mental life.   A scientific cerebral phrenology has thus replaced the doctrine of cranial bumps and excrescences, which was advocated so strenuously by Gall and Spurzheim seventy-five years ago, and which impressed so many of our fathers.   Yet there is still much unknown territory lying within the skull, and cerebral geography offers to the intrepid explorer prizes of infinitely greater importance to the human race than those won, however gallantly, by Nansen, Scott, and Peary.

In this rapid and very incomplete sketch of the structure and functions of the normal human body, I have endeavored to give to you something of the spirit of modern physiology and to impress you with the variety and complexity of our bodily machine.   Unless one learns it step by step one may be overwhelmed with the intricacy of it all.   We should bear in mind that the intricacies of both structure and function are the result of a long evolution.   Of the mode of origin of the earliest rudiments of organs we can only speculate, but it may conceivably have been a more rapid process than their subsequent change into complicated mechanisms.   Locomotion, even in the unicellular forms, required contractile protoplasm.   When the primitive organism became so large that it could not obtain sufficient food by direct absorption from its environment, it may have been a simple matter to infold and produce a primitive alimentary canal.   A simple system of tubes permeating the body and containing a nutrient

c

liquid soon followed. A simple method of nervous communication between the parts originated early, and along with
it certain simple sense-organs. Thus in the more simple of
the cœlenterates we find muscular, alimentary, circulatory,
and nervous systems already begun, and ready for the subsequent long process of development. Within the walls of the
circulatory system a localized aggregation of muscle cells
formed a simple heart. An extension of the surface tissues
became a respiratory gill. Glands secreting digestive ferments
appeared in connection with the alimentary canal. Other
glands communicating with the surface of the body carried
off waste products. An aggregation of neurones performed
the simple function of a primitive brain. Nerves were multi-
plied, and nervous functions became more diverse. New
sense-organs appeared, by which the organism could acquaint
itself with the various forms of energy in the external world.
A change from the original aquatic to a terrestrial life involved
the appearance of lungs and other profound transformations.
Simultaneously with the ever increasing complexity of structure came physiological differentiation and physiological
integration — the greater the differences within the body, the
greater became the correlation between the parts. And so,
step by step, through ages of trial, now advancing, now
receding, the intricacies of form and function that we find
most completely developed in man's body slowly appeared.

In surveying the working of a human body there is one
topic which has been of absorbing interest to physiologists,
physicians, and philosophers of all ages, and at the present
time, with its many systems of mental healing, is much
attracting the attention of the lay public. This is the problem of mind, its nature, the relation of mind and body, and
the possibility of their mutual influence. To consider this

topic is to enter a field of many and diverse opinions, where speculation has always been rife, where experimentation is difficult, and where superlative uncertainty is still supreme. To the naïve thinker, mind and body are two distinct entities, different in nature — the one spiritual, the other material — and each capable of existing and acting apart from the other, and of inducing, modifying, and arresting activity in the other. To the physiologist this view presents insurmountable difficulties. Neither introspection nor extrinsic observation nor laboratory experimentation reveals to him a mind outside a nervous system. He associates human consciousness only with the cortex of a human cerebrum, and only when the cortical neurones are active, — in sleep and other forms of unconsciousness mind no longer exists, except when dreams interpose their feeble and fantastic images. Every mental phenomenon has its neural counterpart, although the vast majority of neural processes are devoid of a mental accompaniment. It is a favorite attitude of physiologists thus to look upon mind as a sign of brain activity, as only one of the several phenomena by which cerebral neurones manifest their activity, albeit mind seems more mysterious than the phenomena which we call physical, such as changes in temperature, in electrical state, and in chemical composition, all of which are manifest when brain cells act. This hypothesis does not postulate the nature of mind, but it regards mind as an accessory phenomenon, or epiphenomenon, and not as the supreme inhabitant of the cerebral protoplasm. If this hypothesis be true, we must alter our naïve ideas concerning the interaction of body and mind. Thus bodily changes may modify mental action, but only by modifying brain action. So, too, the brain through the nerves may modify bodily action. But the mind itself, a sign of brain activity, cannot influence matter, and thus can never be the directing agency of either brain or body. All supposed influence of the mind over the body is thus reduced to brain influence, which, however, may be mirrored in mental acts. Such an hypothesis, whatever its future, appears to me to be the most fruitful working hypothesis for the physiologist at the present time, and it would appear to clarify the now puzzling field of psychotherapy.

We ought not to leave the consideration of the activities of the human body without a glance, however brief, at the problem of the nature of vital actions in general and their control. From the beginning of human speculation — and that means from the beginning of the human race — down to the era of modern science, when speculation has been forced to give way to demonstration, it was thought that a peculiar power resided in the body which was immediately responsible for bodily actions. This power was variously believed to be material and immaterial. The doctrine which lived longest was that of the pneuma, or spirits, which were conceived as matter in an extremely tenuous state, permeating the body and directing the grosser matter of which the body is composed. The Greek physicians, five hundred years before Christ, believed in the spirits, as did their successors in both Greece and Rome. All through the Middle Ages the spirits held sway, but after the Renaissance had set men free from slavish tradition, there entered doubts and a lack of agreement as to what constitutes the directing power in vital actions. Various immaterial agencies were then invoked — the anima or soul, the archeus, the ether, the nervous principle. But these in turn gave way with the advent of a final form of the general doctrine. This was the hypothesis that vital actions are manifestations of a specific force, differing from the forces of inorganic nature, but peculiar to living things, and hence called vital force. The belief in a vital force was almost universal from about the middle of the eighteenth to the middle of the nineteenth century. But toward the end of the period the great advance of physics and chemistry and the application of the new discoveries to living processes profoundly shook the existing belief in regard to the nature of vital phenomena, and led, by the middle of the last century, to the practical abandonment of the doctrine of vitalism. Thus ended the endeavors to explain vital actions by means of a single mysterious principle, and men turned their attention to the discovery of the physical and chemical phenomena, which were, and are still, recognized as the essence of the manifestation of life. The question of vitalism or mechanism is not yet beyond the sphere of debate, but the mechanistic mode of interpreting the phenomena of nature has proved to be the one under which the most rapid progress in discovery has yet been made. One of the scientific features of modern medicine, therefore, is no longer to regard the human body as a thing of mystery, which will forever be inexplicable, but to believe that every part of it, sooner or later, will give up its secrets — to the same extent at least that non-living nature will yield hers.

II

In the last lecture I endeavored to present a picture of the human body in a state of health, healthy as to both structure and function.   To-night I intend to devote the hour to a subject which is popularly less inviting, but to the man of science not less interesting, namely, that of the body in the throes of disease.   By disease we customarily mean that condition in which bodily function or bodily structure exhibits a deviation from what has come to be regarded as the normal. A distinction is sometimes made between structural and functional diseases, the former being those that are characterized by abnormalities of structure, the latter those in which structural abnormalities are wanting.   However convenient such a distinction may be, it is bound, I think, to be dispensed with in the course of time and of increased knowledge, for it is impossible to believe that a condition of altered function can exist, which does not simultaneously involve an alteration of anatomical or chemical structure.   Our present knowledge, however, is not sufficient to demonstrate such alteration in all diseases.

The most universal phenomenon of disease, therefore, is perturbed or altered function.   No sharp line can be drawn between the normal and the diseased.   There are wide and indefinite limits of variation in the working of bodily organs, and it is usually only when the extreme limits are passed and the changed condition continues that it is called pathological.

Thus, the heart of an adult man in middle life beats usually with a perfectly regular rhythm and at an average rate of seventy-two times in the minute; but there may at times be a temporary irregularity or a considerable slowing or quickening without the presence of disease. The bodily temperature, the average of which, when measured in the mouth cavity, is about 98.4° F. in the healthy adult, has a normal daily variation of one and one half degrees or more, and only when it rises to a considerable height or sinks to a considerable depth and there remains, do we suspect anything abnormal.

Disease rarely involves a single function alone. When the alteration of one function has passed beyond the limits of the normal, it is almost certain to carry others in its train. Thus, if the valve between the left auricle and the left ventricle of the heart leaks and becomes incapable of closing the orifice between the two chambers, the onward movement of the blood is interfered with; the lungs may become gorged with blood; and this engorgement may reach backward to the right side of the heart and the veins of the body generally. At the same time too little blood may pass on from the left ventricle to the arteries. The results may be far-reaching. The heart muscle may become increased in quantity in the endeavor to compensate for the circulatory disturbance by a more powerful beat. The heart may, however, suffer from palpitation, weakness, and irregularity. The person may be distressed from lack of the proper respiratory exchange of oxygen and carbonic acid. Bronchitis, cough, and hemorrhage from the lungs may occur. The cavities of the chest and the abdomen may become partially filled with liquid that has exuded from the blood. The legs may likewise become œdematous from the same reason. There may be nausea and loss of appetite, and digestion in the stomach may be interfered with. The liver may become congested; blood may escape into its tissues and its cells may undergo atrophy, while its various functions may be seriously deranged. And lastly, the kidneys may perform their work only in part.

From this involvement of other organs besides the primarily diseased one it follows that a disease may often be an affair of very great complexity. We often speak of the symptoms of a disease as if they were to be distinguished from the thing that gives rise to them. The word "symptoms" is used, rather loosely, to signify the more obvious signs of the disease. If, however, we should employ the word in a strict sense, as including all the pathological phenomena, symptoms and disease would be synonymous terms, the disease being nothing more or less than the sum of its symptoms or manifestations. Just as normal function is now regarded as a matter of chemistry and physics, so is disease; the symptoms of disease being changed chemical or physical conditions. Disease is not, therefore, a specific entity, a thing, arising spontaneously within the body or entering it from without. It is merely a change from what has come to be regarded as the normal.

But this modern conception has not always been the accepted one, and a most interesting chapter in human history is that which deals with the views that have been held respecting the nature and causation of disease. As might be expected, these views have been many and various. According to the earliest known and a very persistent conception, disease is a demon or strange spirit, which has invaded the body and causes it to perform new and unwonted actions. This view was held by the Sumerian predecessors of the Babylonians, by the Babylonians themselves, and by later peoples, and it is still found among primitive races.

With some peoples the demon is the spirit of a human being, who has lived and died, and whose ghost returns to inhabit again for a period a living body. This theory of demoniac possession was widespread among the Jewish races at the time of Christ, and the casting out of devils was a common method of healing. Christ himself not only drove such evil or unclean spirits out of the body, but he said of those who believed in him, "In my name shall they cast out devils." Even down to quite recent times civilized people have believed in demoniac possession, especially by those suffering from mental or nervous diseases. Allied to this is the belief in witches, and although it has been more than two hundred years since the last witch was hanged at Salem, this strange delusion has probably not yet died out among the ignorant of our land.

From time immemorial, by both the adherents and the opponents of the demoniac theory of disease, endeavors have been made to find an explanation in natural or material agencies. The first to do this in a really effective manner was an eminent Greek physician, Hippocrates by name, who lived in the fifth century before Christ. The title of "Father of Medicine" has been given to Hippocrates by those system-loving historians who find satisfaction in ascribing to single individuals the paternity of great sciences. This title is deserved not so much by reason of the original contributions which Hippocrates made, as because he and his contemporaries present, in the large body of Hippocratic writings, a graphic and stimulating picture of the best medicine of their time. The Hippocratic writers upheld nobly the ideals of the medical vocation. They assumed to exist within the body four cardinal fluids, or "humors," which they called respectively blood, phlegm, yellow bile, and black bile. Health is present when the humors exist in proper quantities and proper relations to one another; disease when the proper quantities and relations are disturbed. This was the beginning of the so-called humoral pathology and of an academic controversy, which has raged for twenty-three hundred years and the echoes of which have not wholly died away, between those who ascribe disease to the fluids and those who ascribe it to the solids of the body, the humoralists and the solidists. The humoral hypothesis has stamped itself indelibly in popular speech. While not subscribing to the Hippocratic pathology we may be good-humored or bad-humored; the melancholy person is suffering from black bile, the choleric person from yellow bile; and he who possesses a phlegmatic or a sanguine temperament derives it from the excess of his cardinal phlegm or blood.

Hippocrates and his followers, among whom ought to be especially mentioned the great Roman physician Galen of the second century before Christ, did not, however, ascribe all disease solely to the faults of the humors; for the peccadilloes of the pneuma had still to be reckoned with, the extremely subtile material spirits, which were believed to be largely responsible for bodily actions. From the time of Pericles and Sophocles and Praxiteles down to that of Charles I, Harvey, and Descartes, a heavy burden of disease was laid upon the humors and the spirits. But even these two thousand years of supremacy could not prevent the investigators of the Renaissance from having discourteous doubts about the importance and even the existence of these two agents. One of the first of the doubters was Paracelsus, who had alchemistic tendencies and who was bold and illogical enough to displace the humors with still more hypothetical substances, symbolically termed "sulphur, mercury and salt," and the pneuma with the equally mysterious "archeus." The stomach was the seat of the archeus, and if it did not perform its duties properly, disease resulted. It was also a favorite notion of the time that diseases were sent by God as a punishment for the sins of man. "Ira Dei" as a cause of disease has perhaps not yet wholly disappeared from some circles, even though it is not met with in the clinic and the reports of the board of health. Further causes were sought in supposed "fermentations," "stoppages" within the blood-vessels or nerves, and various mysterious dynamic agencies. All these strange ideas culminated in the "vital force" of a century ago. But with the great extension of the scientific mode of thought and the increase of scientific knowledge that occurred during the first half of the nineteenth century, which were marked among other things by the rise of the science of biology, pathological doctrine underwent a profound change. Men of medicine saw the futility of attempting to explain all diseases by means of a common principle; "systems" were done away with; uncontrolled speculation and deductive reasoning from hypothetical assumptions were replaced by laboratory and clinical observations; and modern scientific medicine, with its conception of disease as altered function, accompanied by more or less obvious alteration of structure, was born.

Pathological alterations of structure and function may be innumerable. To illustrate their possibilities let me enumerate some of the various disorders that may befall two of the body's organs, the heart and the liver; the one in which physical, the other in which chemical, phenomena predominate.

The heart's muscular walls may become unduly increased in thickness, owing to excessive growth of its muscular tissue.

Its muscle cells may become separated from one another, or torn into fragments, or their substance may be replaced in part by fat or chalky material or other useless substances; this may lead to weakening and even rupture of the heart walls. The connective tissue within the walls may become the seat of harmful changes; tumors may develop therein. The arteries supplying the walls with blood may become closed by particles cast off from other diseased organs, and this in turn may lead to degeneration of the heart tissue. The pericardium, or membrane surrounding the heart, may become the seat of dangerous inflammation or other affections. The heart's cavities may become unduly dilated. The endocardium, or membrane lining the heart's walls, may undergo inflammatory changes and become the seat of foreign growths associated with the presence of bacteria. The same events may occur in the valves, which may also become thickened, hardened, or otherwise deformed. They may become incapable of adequately closing, and thus regurgitations of the blood from one cavity to another, or from the arteries to the heart, may occur; in this way the onward progress of the blood may be seriously interfered with. The openings between the heart chambers, or between the chambers and the arteries may become narrow, and thus again the progress of the blood may be hindered. The heart beats may become unduly slowed or quickened, or augmented or weakened in force; they may occur irregularly, owing to a variety of causes; the chambers may possess different rhythms. The terrible pain of angina may occur. There may exist various malformations of the heart which date from fœtal life, and seriously incapacitate the organ for meeting adult conditions. And, lastly, this all-important organ is subject, like other organs, to wounds and other external injuries.

These are some of the more pronounced abnormalities in one of the body's organs. Probably there are many others which are still obscure. The careful observation and experimentation of the future will reveal them.

Let me here interpolate a warning against a possible danger. It is a rather common tendency of the introspective human mind, when contemplating the picture of a disease, to transfer its details to one's own person. You have perhaps heard of the author into whose hands there once fell a book on diseases, and who was sufficiently bedevilled by it to read it through. As he proceeded, to his growing horror he found that one by one he possessed in his own body the successive symptoms, and at the end of the book he came to realize that he was the victim of each and every malady therein described — except one, which went by the plain English name of "housemaid's knee," whatever that may mean. I have a medical friend whose name is well known among men of science, and who rarely investigates a disease without coming to believe that he himself suffers from it. Each disease remains until it is duly displaced by the next in the course of his researches. I trust that you will not leave this hall to-night with the belief that your own hearts are affected by the many disorders that I have just enumerated.

The heart's functions are primarily mechanical, and correspondingly its diseases are manifested chiefly by mechanical phenomena. With other organs, such, for example, as the liver, chemical phenomena predominate both in health and disease. The diseases of the liver are characterized anatomically by various forms of degeneration or death of the liver cells; increase in its connective tissue; the appearance of abscesses, cancer, and other tumors; various inflammatory, catarrhal, or other conditions of the bile ducts, which obstruct the outflow of bile and may lead to its passage into the blood — a condition which is known as jaundice; inflammation of the gall bladder; the appearance therein of gall stones; various affections of the hepatic blood-vessels and lymphatic vessels, and, lastly, injuries or malformations, a common cause of which is tight lacing. As might be expected, these structural abnormalities are associated with functional disturbances. The capacity of the liver to store up starch and to feed the body's tissues may be interfered with; the production of bile, with whatever that fluid means to digestion and the absorption of food, may be diminished; the elimination of harmful waste matters may be lessened, with a resultant overloading of the organism with them; and various poisonous substances may pass on to the tissues without receiving their customary detoxication. Experiment seems to show that some of these disorders may occur without harmful results to the individual, but most of them are, in all probability, seriously detrimental.

This brief enumeration of some of the diseases to which two of the essential organs of the body are subject, will prove sufficient, I trust, to give you some notion of "the thousand natural shocks that flesh is heir to." In thinking of them, moreover, we should bear in mind what I have previously said, that any one of them is rarely limited to the primary seat of the disease, but is practically certain to involve other organs and other functions. And herein lies much of the seriousness of any pathological state, while this fact, moreover, increases the difficulties of the physician.

Because of our ignorance of the nature and cause of many maladies no classification of diseases that has yet been proposed is altogether satisfactory. The following list includes some of the main groups of human diseases : —

(1) Infectious diseases; *e.g.* typhoid fever, smallpox, tuberculosis, diphtheria.

(2) Poisoning; *e.g.* alcoholism, morphia habit, lead poisoning.

(3) Constitutional diseases ; *e.g.* rheumatism, gout, diabetes.

(4) Diseases of organs.

When a physician is called upon to treat a case of illness, the first task that confronts him is that of determining the nature and the primary seat of the disease. His success in treatment must presuppose a correct diagnosis. Here his troubles begin. If his patient were a non-living machine, whose mechanism could be readily taken apart and whose parts could be separately examined, repaired, cleaned, lubricated, tested, and replaced, the location and nature of the disease might be readily discovered and a cure might be readily effected. But he has no such easy task. His patient is a living, sentient, human body, endowed with the most mysterious of all qualities, whose members cannot at will be removed and returned to their places, and whose secrets are largely hidden from even the most careful observation. Through only a few avenues are these secrets revealed. From the beginning of the human race these avenues have not changed, and it is one of the great achievements of modern scientific medicine that along them have been found innumerable clues of which physicians of even a century ago had no conception. Scientific diagnosis, though it is still far from the ideal and still finds itself too often mistaken, has in recent years made great strides. This is due largely to the fact that exact physical and chemical methods for detecting disease have come into use. From the earliest healing down to about the beginning of the nineteenth century, physicians had few means of diagnosis except those of the unaided senses. Sounds and specula had occasionally been employed for exploring some of the body's orifices. There were men in advance of their time who had applied the thermometer to the skin for determining bodily temperature, and the watch had likewise been used for counting the pulse. But most physicians were content to observe the patient and question him, feel his skin and his pulse, watch the blood which they freely drew from his veins, and observe certain of his excreta. It was inevitable that much skill and cleverness in interpreting the symptoms thus observed had become developed, but it is obvious that advance was painfully slow.

A really valuable contribution to diagnostic aids was made by a medical practitioner of Vienna, named Auenbrugger, who had learned that the resonance of the chest was modified by disease. In order to determine the degree of this resonance he proposed the method of percussion, or gentle tapping of the chest walls. But it was not until well after the beginning of the nineteenth century that under French influence this method was perfected and extended to the many viscera of the chest and the abdomen.

Although the ear had previously been employed for listening to certain internal sounds, it was not until 1815 that Laennec, a Parisian physician, devised the stethoscope, by which the sounds caused by the beating of the heart, the passage of the air to and from the lungs, and other internal movements can be heard. This was the beginning of the invaluable method of auscultation. Oliver Wendell Holmes, who had the good fortune to study medicine in Paris, was one of the first in this country to recognize the value of the new discovery, and in 1836 won a prize offered for the best dissertation on "How far are the external means of exploring the condition of the internal organs to be considered useful and important in medical practice?" Dr. Holmes' success, however, did not prevent him from writing also his far less serious poem entitled, "The Stethoscope Song," in which his scientific hero, fresh from the Parisian clinics, came to grief because of the strange diagnoses he made through the aid of his new-fangled instrument, in which "a couple of very impertinent" and very buzzy flies had chanced to make their abode. The stethoscope has gradually undergone improvements, and to-day is the indispensable aid of every physician. Through the addition to it of a microphone and a delicate galvanometer it has recently become possible to make permanent photographic records of physiological sounds, and thus to make detailed analyses of them.

Equally indispensable has become the clinical thermometer for the exact determination of bodily temperatures, especially in fevers. Its universal introduction was likewise one of the achievements of the last century.

Of great value also was the ingenious invention of the ophthalmoscope in 1851, by the German physicist, Helmholtz. This instrument made possible for the first time the illumination of the interior of the eyeball, and thus facilitated, not only a physical examination of that organ, but through it the detection of certain constitutional diseases. The principle of internal illumination has been extended, until there are few organs possessing external orifices that cannot thus be explored. The latest achievement by means of illumination, the echoes of whose initial success have not yet died away, is the discovery by Roentgen of the penetrating power of the X- or Roentgen rays. These rays, transmitted by certain tissues and held back by others, are now used, not only for

D

localizing foreign bodies, such as bullets, and in the study of the bones, but also for the observation of pathological conditions in various other organs, such as the heart, the lungs and the stomach.

The labors of physiologists to determine the facts of the circulation of the blood have been richly productive for pathology and practical medicine. These labors are now coming to fruition in the matter of diagnosis. The heart's activity is accessible to observation through various devices. I have already referred to the stethoscope, which is used in transmitting heart sounds either to the ear or to a photographic plate. Like other organs, the heart in action constitutes an electric battery, and with each beat its different parts are the seat of differences in electrical potential. These differences may be detected even on the surface of the body by a delicate galvanometer. The instrument most commonly used contains an excessively fine thread of quartz or platinum, suspended between magnets. When two points on the surface of the body, such as two hands, or a hand and a foot, are placed in circuit with the thread, it bends from side to side with each heart beat. These motions may be photographed, and thus an exact, graphic record may be obtained of the electrical changes involved in the heart's action. Normal hearts make normal records. Pathological hearts make records corresponding to their abnormalities, and thus a new clue is obtained to the presence and the nature of diseased conditions. That this method is not merely a scientific curiosity is proved by the fact that it is now being introduced into hospitals and clinics as a practical diagnostic aid. It is not necessary that the galvanometer be in the immediate presence of the patient. Accurate records of the heart beat have been transmitted through electric wires for at least one mile and a half.

Columbia University Lectures

SCIENTIFIC FEATURES OF MODERN MEDICINE

THE JESUP LECTURES

1911

COLUMBIA
UNIVERSITY PRESS
SALES AGENTS
NEW YORK:
LEMCKE & BUECHNER
30–32 WEST 27TH STREET
LONDON:
HENRY FROWDE
AMEN CORNER, E.C.
TORONTO:
HENRY FROWDE
25 RICHMOND ST., W.

COLUMBIA UNIVERSITY LECTURES

SCIENTIFIC FEATURES OF MODERN MEDICINE

BY

FREDERIC S. LEE, Ph.D.

DALTON PROFESSOR OF PHYSIOLOGY, COLUMBIA UNIVERSITY

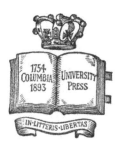

New York

THE COLUMBIA UNIVERSITY PRESS

1911

Norwood Press
J. S. Cushing Co. — Berwick & Smith Co.
Norwood, Mass., U.S.A.

The beat of the heart can be readily observed through various movements of the surface of the body. The most widely recognized of these movements is that of the pulse, which is the wavelike impulse given by the heart in its contractions to the blood in the arteries. The pulse can be detected in many arteries, but most conveniently in the radial artery of the wrist, where it not only can be felt by the finger, but often causes a perceptible rise and fall of the surface of the skin. The heart beats are also appreciable in the jugular veins, which lie near the surface at the neck; while the muscular walls of the chest on the left side between the fifth and sixth ribs and outside the lower end of the heart receive an impulse directly from the heart itself. Nearly fifty years ago a French physiologist, Marey, devised a delicate instrument by which these various movements can be magnified by a lever and be recorded in a graphic manner on paper. This instrument he called the sphygmograph, which means literally "wave writer," and its self-written record is the sphygmogram. From the records of these various movements much can be learned regarding the physical condition and movements of the heart and arteries and their state of health or disease. The difficulties of interpreting the details of sphygmograms, which are great and have not yet been wholly removed, and the large amount of experience that is required with the instrument, have prevented its universal use.

Another instrument for the exact study of the condition of the blood-circulatory system, however, is winning favor. Through the investigations of physiologists on the bodies of animals, it is known that the blood exists in the arteries under a considerable degree of pressure. The amount of this pressure depends on the force of the heart beat, the physical characteristics of the arterial walls, the degree of resistance to the blood flow that is offered by the small arteries and capillaries, and other factors. The walls of the arteries are richly provided with nerves, through which a particular portion of the brain can control the caliber of the vessels and thus can control in some degree the pressure of the blood. This system of nervous control is known as the vasomotor system. We recognize a vasomotor center in the brain, and two kinds of vasomotor nerves, called respectively vasoconstrictor and vasodilator. The caliber of the arteries and therewith the blood pressure in a particular part of the body can be altered through the vasomotor nervous mechanism in accordance with the amount of blood required by that part at a given time. The system is very perfectly organized and works with a degree of exactness that might be expected of a mechanism that has taken many thousands, or even millions, of years to become perfected. The blood pressure varies not only with varying physiological states, but with a great variety of diseased conditions as well. It is obvious that a determination of the degree of blood pressure affords valuable insight into the internal mechanism of the body and its varying conditions. Early in the eighteenth century the Reverend Stephen Hales, rector of a country parish in the south of England, was possessed of a curiosity to investigate many odd and unknown things in nature. Among other strange achievements, he succeeded in measuring the pressure exerted by the blood in the arteries of the horse. This experiment, singular as it must have seemed to his unscientific contemporaries, was the forerunner of great things. Through the perfection of vivisectional methods it has since been possible to make very exact determinations of arterial pressure in animals, but it is only during the past fifteen years that means have been found by which similar determinations are possible in the intact bodies of living human beings. Instruments, called sphygmomanometers, now exist which can be taken directly to the bedside, and by which the accurate measurement of the blood pressure in the patient's arteries can be quickly made. The use of such instruments reveals that inferences regarding the state of the blood-circulatory organs, which are drawn from feeling the throbbing artery with the unaided finger, may be inexact and often quite misleading. The advantages of the new method are so great that the intelligent physician can hardly fail to add the new applicance to his constantly increasing equipment.

I have mentioned but a few of the instruments of precision of which the modern physician makes use. The list might be indefinitely extended to include the elaborate electrical appliances, by means of which the irritability of muscles and nerves, paralysis, and many other affections of the nervous system are detected, the various instruments for testing the delicacy of sight, hearing, and other special senses, and so on. I had almost forgotten to speak of the microscope, without which modern medical practice would be impossible. The universal use of the microscope as an aid to diagnosis was made possible by the discovery of a method of eliminating the color effects due to the chromatic aberration of the early lenses. Efficient achromatic objectives were first made in the third decade of the nineteenth century. With their aid the physician recognizes disease germs and the characteristics of diseased tissues, numbers the corpuscles of the blood, and in innumerable ways augments many thousand fold the powers of his unaided eye.

If the twentieth-century diagnostician has thus become a physicist, he is perhaps even more a chemist. Physiological chemistry or biochemistry is largely the growth ·of a single generation, but its accumulations are exceedingly abundant, and they have been promptly utilized for the service of medicine.   We now know much concerning the play of the atoms and molecules within the body and how they misbehave during disease.   These activities, both normal and pathological, are reflected especially in the various liquids which are contained within the body or are given off from it.   The blood and the urine are the most significant of these for diagnostic purposes.   With both of these liquids both chemical and physical abnormalities frequently signify, not merely that the liquids themselves, or the organs that are immediately concerned in their preparation, are at fault, but that organs or tissues remotely concerned with their preparation are abnormal.   Moreover, they often indicate, in addition to the specific diseases of specific organs, more general metabolic diseases.

While the days of medieval blood-letting are fortunately passed, it has been found that even a few drops of blood, following the pricking of the skin by a needle, are sufficient to give clues to the presence of a considerable number of maladies.   The determination of the amount of hemoglobin, the red coloring matter of the blood, or of the number of red corpuscles, is valuable in detecting such affections as the various forms of anemia, which in turn may be indicative of the presence of other diseases.   The amount of hemoglobin present in the blood of anemic individuals may be only fifteen or twenty per cent of the normal amount.   Mere pallor of the skin, which may be present in anemia, may also be due to other causes and does not necessarily indicate an anemic condition.   The average number of leucocytes in one cubic millimeter of the blood of healthy persons varies between 5000 and 10,000. In certain diseases it may far exceed these figures, in others it may be far less. Thus, in pneumonia the number of leucocytes is frequently as many as 40,000 or more, while in typhoid fever there is usually a diminution below the normal. The relative frequence of the several varieties of the corpuscles is also significant. Bacteria and other parasites are frequently found in blood. It has recently been discovered that the blood serum of persons suffering from typhoid fever, when added to a liquid containing living typhoid germs, causes the latter to cease moving and to aggregate together in crowds. This peculiar phenomenon is the basis of a new test for the presence of typhoid, the Widal test, which has proved a most valuable addition to diagnostic methods. One of the greatest advances has been along the lines of the new physical chemistry. The degree of molecular concentration of the blood, or, in other words, the relative number of molecules and ions contained within it, is significant. Recent work has shown that this can be determined by the comparatively simple procedure of observing at what temperature the serum, or liquid portion of clotted blood, freezes. Healthy blood serum freezes at approximately $-.56°$ C., *i.e.* half a degree lower than the point at which pure water freezes. If, however, the freezing point is found to be lower than the normal, the blood contains too large a proportion of solids, and the inference is justified that the kidneys are not performing their full function.

While the physical and chemical characteristics of the urine constitute the key to certain maladies of the kidneys, their significance reaches far beyond that organ, by reason of the fact that the urine represents a most important medium, in which the tissues of the whole body eliminate both normal and abnormal material. There are few tissues which do not exhibit through the urine their functional peculiarities. Not only the kidneys, but the liver, the heart, the muscles, the digestive and other organs, thus reflect their state of health or disease. A most elaborate science has therefore grown up around the study of this one product of bodily activity. Of significance as diagnostic aids are the amount of the urine; its specific gravity; its freezing point and hence its molecular concentration; its color; its acid or alkaline reaction; its content in nitrogen, as well as urea, uric acid, various proteins, pigments, sugars, and other organic compounds, as well as various inorganic constituents; and the presence of blood, of crystals of various kinds, of bacteria, of body cells and of "casts," a pathological product, visible to the microscope, and formed in the minute secreting tubes of the kidney.

However skillful diagnosis has become, it often makes mistakes. It often happens that derangements do not reveal themselves until long after they ought to be attended to. Now and then the combination of symptoms simulates something different from that which is really present. At times the best of doctors disagree as to the interpretation of symptoms. A well-known and learned American physician has recently published results of a courageous study of mistaken diagnoses, which was based on a comparison of the conditions as indicated by clinical observations and the conditions as actually revealed by the autopsies of the same patients. It is a valuable contribution to the literature of medical errors. At the same time it reveals the present hopeful attitude of the best of the medical profession. The physician has never before appreciated so keenly the necessity of correct diagnosis. If in the past he has done those things which he ought not to have done, and confessed his faults in the proper spirit of humiliation and repentance, his mistakes hereafter will be fewer in number. And they are daily becoming fewer. The sharp, critical analysis of diseased conditions and their prompt detection are two of the prominent features of modern medicine, and largely contribute to its right to be called scientific.

III

METHODS OF TREATING DISEASE

In the two previous lectures we have considered normal structure and function and some of their perturbations in disease. We are continually beset by agencies, powers of pathological darkness, without and within, which, if unopposed, would turn us from the straight and narrow path of health and lead us into chaos. We may oppose these evil agencies in two ways: either through our innate powers of resistance, or by recourse to the help which medical science offers. In the present lecture I wish to consider these two methods of combating disease.

Physicians used to speak of the *vis medicatrix naturæ*, the healing power of nature. The phrase expressed an idea as mystical as that of *vis vitalis*. We no longer use the words, but the principle persists. Modern medicine has analyzed it and now terms it the natural defenses of the organism against disease. Darwin has drawn a graphic picture of the struggle that, to preserve their existence, living organisms wage against other living organisms. Every variation in structure or function that gives one the advantage over another tends by so much toward the preservation of the one and the destruction of the other. Nature is ever selecting her favorites and endowing them with special gifts. They survive, while their rivals perish. By the inheritance and accumulation of beneficial variations the organism becomes constantly more complex and better adapted to cope with the conditions of existence. Fifty years after the publication of the "Origin of Species" biology is questioning in how far natural selection is a factor in organic change. But whatever the cause, the fact is not to be denied that in the course of evolution the internal mechanisms of organisms have become more efficient in meeting the many vicissitudes to which they are subject. Accidents and disease are prominent among these vicissitudes, and against them organisms are provided with many natural means of defense. It is worth our while, I think, to consider these provisions of nature, before going on to discuss the various artificial agencies which man makes use of in his fight against disease.

Nature has been generous to the human race. With eyes, ears, hands, lungs, kidneys, and various other glands she has given us a double equipment, and even if one organ of each pair be lost, the cripple's powers of life are not seriously impaired. Tuberculosis may destroy one lung, and the other, if it be healthy, will take in oxygen and give out carbonic acid in the same quantities which formerly passed through the two organs together. The surgeon knows that if to save a patient's life, he must remove a diseased kidney, the other kidney, if healthy, will at once begin to perform the functions of both, and with rapid growth in size and amount of secreting tissue, will soon become capable of double labor. It has recently been shown that the thyroids and the adrenal bodies are profoundly related to certain bodily processes. The total removal of thyroid tissue causes serious physical and mental abnormalities, yet these are obviated if even one fifth of the tissue is left. The total removal of both the adrenal bodies is followed by speedy death, but serious results are averted if even a mere fragment of one be left. Similar lavish generosity of tissue is exhibited by unpaired organs. Surgical experiments on animals have shown that in them one half or three fourths of the liver and nine tenths of the pancreas may be removed without endangering life. Surgeons have removed from man's body without fatal results, parts of or even the entire stomach, or considerable portions of the intestine. Certain portions of the brain which control certain bodily movements may be removed without the serious impairment of these movements, since other portions of the brain seem to be capable of performing the work of the lost parts. Nearly one half of the blood may be lost without permanently serious effects. In certain cases similar labors are carried on by anatomically different organs, and the loss of one does not mean that the body is wholly deprived of the common function. Thus if a person closes his eyes and attempts to walk, he will be dizzy and uncertain in his movements. This simple experiment teaches him that customarily his eyes are an aid in the maintenance of his bodily equilibrium. With blind persons other senses must perform the entire work of indicating to the brain the equilibrium needs of the body. Both the stomach and the pancreas produce ferments that are capable of digesting proteins, and the salivary glands and the pancreas others that digest starches.

Allied to these instances of the generosity of nature are cases of adaptability to changed conditions. In accordance with our bodily needs our heart beats rapidly or slowly; we breathe more or less rapidly and more or less deeply — thus in fever we automatically breathe rapidly and thus endeavor to keep down our abnormal temperature; our various arteries become constricted or dilated; we contract our muscles to a greater or a less degree; we use for mechanical purposes more or less of the energy of our food; we produce and eliminate more or less heat — if we are cold, we shiver to

PREFACE

An appointment to the lectureship founded by an appreciative and generous patron of science, the late Morris K. Jesup, Esq., has given me an opportunity to present some of the striking features of modern medicine which illustrate its genuinely scientific character, its great change from the medicine of the past, and its hopeful outlook for the future. Obviously no attempt could here be made to survey its whole field; but I have endeavored, through a consideration of selected topics, to depict its spirit. Human beings may be divided into those who do, and those who do not, believe in the efficiency of medicine. The relative number of nonbelievers has always been small, and is doubtless much less now than in the days of the Greeks and of Molière, but their sentiments have ever been loudly proclaimed. It is hoped that these pages may be read by both classes. They may perchance help to fortify the believers, and, if not actually to convert the dissenters, at least to make their doubts appear less rational. The labors of a learned profession can easily be belittled by those who are less learned. I shall be gratified if what I have here written shall be instrumental in inducing laymen to study the human body and appreciate what men of medicine are now doing to maintain health and to prevent, diagnose, treat, and cure disease. When laymen do this, the influence of medical cults and healing sects is sure to decline.

The lectures here published were delivered at the American Museum of Natural History in the city of New York during the months of February and March, 1911. As with previous lectures on the same foundation, the endeavor has been to present the subject matter clear-cut and in language that is

not too technical for the intelligent layman.   The latter
is often eager to learn, but cannot be criticised if he finds the
literature of science written in words that are foreign to his
mother tongue.   In a few cases I have taken the liberty of
quoting from previous writings of my own, without acknowl-
edging the repetition of my language.   It has been found
impracticable to reproduce the many illustrations that were
helpful in the oral presentation of the lectures.

My thanks are due to my colleagues, Professors Francis
Carter Wood and Phillip Hanson Hiss, and Drs. W. A. Bas-
tedo and H. H. Janeway, and to other friends, Drs. Simon
Flexner, William Hallock Park, James Ewing, Alexis Carrel,
Nathan W. Green, and Major F. F. Russell.   Several of these
friends have read critically portions of my manuscript and
have offered helpful suggestions.

FREDERIC S. LEE.

COLUMBIA UNIVERSITY,
    October 1, 1911.

warm ourselves; and we either oxidize our food at once or store it for future needs. In the course of normal activity we produce various chemical substances which are poisonous to protoplasm and, if allowed to accumulate, would be dangerous to health. Our bodily adaptability is such, however, that our tissues promptly seize upon these substances, and by chemical combination render them innocuous. If bacteria enter the body, the harmful toxins that they give off stimulate our cells to produce antitoxins, and by a union of the two the bacterial products are made harmless; or antibacterial substances are produced, which destroy the invading germs. If a cut in the skin brings the blood, it promptly clots at the wounded spot and further hemorrhage is avoided. The value of this power is sadly demonstrated by those unfortunate persons in whose bodies the essential factors in blood coagulation are wanting, and a trifling wound allows their vital fluid slowly to ooze away.

The natural defenses of the body against disease are nowhere more strikingly shown than in the leucocytes, or white blood corpuscles. It was the French biologist, Metchnikoff, the present sous-directeur of the Pasteur Institute in Paris, who first claimed that the true worth of the leucocytes had never been recognized. In a body suffering from an invasion of bacteria he noticed that many of the microbes were inclosed within the bodies of the white blood cells. He investigated the phenomenon, and was led to the idea that one of the duties of leucocytes is to destroy bacteria, many of which are the germs of diseases, by deliberately engulfing, killing, and digesting them, and thus to protect the body from the foreign invaders. To the cells engaged in this work he gave the name phagocytes, signifying eating cells, and to the process phagocytosis. It is now agreed that Metchnikoff discovered here a phenomenon of wide occurrence and of the greatest value to the individual. To leucocytes, furthermore, have been ascribed the production and elimination of chemical substances which are poisonous to bacteria and kill them without previous ingestion. Thus in two ways are the white blood cells inimical to our organic enemies. Many of them accumulate at the parts of the body which are the natural ports of entry of the foreign cells, such as in the walls of the air passages, along the alimentary canal, and wherever the skin is cut or injured. They there form an advance guard to repel invaders. If this guard is overpowered, there still exists the main force of leucocytes scattered throughout the organism and ready to pounce upon the aliens wherever found — and woe betide the luckless germ that actually enters the tissues! Leucocytes are ever ready to give up their lives to duty, and large numbers are destroyed daily, to be replaced by new ones born in the lymphatic glands and the marrow of the bones. Little do we realize what watchful defenders are constantly, day and night, caring for our personal safety.[1]

I have mentioned but a few of the numerous protective provisions of nature with which our bodies are endowed. Our power of ready and harmonious physiological adaptation to our environment in the interests of ourselves is one of the most valuable of our possessions. It has become customary to deride the idea of teleology, but however unscientific the teleological point of view of a half century ago appears now, the fact of the protective adaptation of organic means to environmental conditions cannot be denied. Through our innate powers our bodies are constantly endeavoring, whether we wish it so or not, to maintain their health

[1] See also pp. 77 and 79.

and ward off disease and death.   We are inclined, I think, to underestimate both the numbers of the hostile agencies surrounding us and our powers of resistance.

But there come times in the experience of all of us when our own powers prove inadequate, and it is then that if we are not beguiled by the seductive words of quackery, we turn for aid to the physician and his science and art.   We can only surmise regarding the beginning of the art of healing, for the earliest historical records give evidence of its preëxistence. Since even animals are known to employ healing methods, as is illustrated by the facts that cats and dogs lick their wounds and monkeys try with their paws to stop a flow of blood, it is probable that primeval man inherited certain curative instincts.   His subsequent medical acquisitions undoubtedly originated largely in empiricism, the experience of individuals in securing relief from pain and physical discomfort.   Crude empiricism indeed has given us a great portion of the medical art down to the nineteenth century, and it has not yet disappeared.   It was early joined by magic, and magic's healthful amulets are still seen in the rabbit's foot and the horseshoe, which ward off witches and bring good luck, and in the potato that is still carried in the pocket to cure rheumatism. In the division of labor among the people of a race the art of healing was early assumed by specific individuals — the savage tribe of the present time has its medicine man.   With the appearance of religions priests took over the art in some degree, but even in early Greek times the medical profession, distinct from the priesthood, existed, and it has gradually acquired a position of constantly increasing authority.

The scientific physician of to-day makes use of, and in so far as he is able, reënforces the patient's natural means of defense.   But he supplements these by a host of agencies, the sum of which in his pedantic moments he is pleased to call his *armamentarium*. Besides the surgical methods he employs for therapeutic purposes drugs, foods, water, serums, vaccines, electricity, heat and cold, mechanical agents, rest, exercise, massage, climate, mental influences, and, in fact, whatever physical, chemical, and psychical agencies seem to be helpful. I shall devote the remainder of this hour to a consideration of some of these measures.

Drugs, which may be of vegetable, animal, or mineral origin, constitute one of the most ancient and universal of all of the material agencies employed by man for his manifold purposes. There never has been a period in human history when they have not been known. They have been celebrated in love potions and as holding the secrets of perpetual youth; in magic and superstition they have been indispensable; in political intrigue they have been potent; and in the treatment of diseases no agent has been more resorted to. Primitive knowledge of the action of drugs was doubtless obtained chiefly from crude empiricism. In the Middle Ages the curious doctrine of "signatures" arose, and its contributions to materia medica are still influential in popular medicine. According to this, the Creator placed signs upon natural objects to indicate to men their uses. Thus, from the fact that the leaflets of *Oxalis* are heart-shaped, it was believed that they were effective in diseases of the heart. The resemblance of the "fibers" of the hepatic, *Marchantia*, to the "fibers" of the liver signified that this plant is to be employed in diseases of the liver, hence the name liverwort. We can trace similar notions in the common plant names, lungwort, kidneywort, and maidenhair. Adder's tongue cured the bites of snakes, and yellow flowers jaundice. A garden was thus full of evidence of God's care of man.

The doctrine was carried to great lengths. The seventeenth-century herbarist, William Coles, author of "Adam in Eden: or Natures Paradiſe," relates that "*Wall-nuts* have the perfect Signature of the Head: The outer husk or green Covering, repreſent the *Pericranium*, or outward skin of the skull, whereon the hair groweth and therefore ſalt made of thoſe husks or barks, are exceeding good for wounds in the head. . . . The *Kernel* hath the very figure of the Brain, and therefore it is very profitable for the Brain, and refiſts poysons; For if the kernel be bruiſed, and moyſtned with the quinteſſence of Wine, and laid upon the Crown of the Head, it comforts the brain and head mightily."

The exact study of the actions of drugs did not begin until the nineteenth century, the first laboratory for their investigation having been established in Dorpat in 1856. In the fifty-five years that have elapsed since then, the science of pharmacology has arisen. The day of "simples" has nearly passed, however much we may regret it who recall our grandmothers' attics with their bundles of smelly herbs. An herb in the attic, it must be confessed, brings up sweeter memories than its decoction, for camomile, spearmint, sage, and hemlock used to send the cold shivers running up and down our little spinal columns. But our grandmothers' simples are really composites. In 1817 morphine was extracted from opium. This was the first of the active principles of drugs to be made known, and now active principles take the place of the former crude mixtures. Other examples of active principles that have been isolated from the crude drugs are strychnine from nux vomica, quinine from cinchona, and atropin from belladonna. Official standards of purity now exist in most civilized countries and are recorded in the national pharmacopeias. Our knowledge of the actions of drugs on living substance has been placed upon an exact basis. Formerly if one wished to know experimentally the action of a drug, he administered it to his fellow-men or, in some cases, to animals, and watched the effect. The great Mithradates, king of Pontus, is said to have been so inconsiderate as to study the actions of poisons upon his relatives, but lest we blacken his character too deeply, it should be added that he also experimented upon them with antidotes. A modern pharmacologist, aware of the extraordinary complexity of the body, realizes that experimentation on the human body is crude and inexact, and therefore proceeds by refined methods, which constantly become more refined and approach ever nearer a mathematical ideal of exactitude, to examine the action of known quantities of the drug on the functions of each of the individual organs or tissues of the animal body, isolated as far as possible from the other organs or tissues. This is supplemented by a similarly exact study of the behavior of combinations of organs or tissues under the influence of the drug. Still further experiments, performed outside of the living tissues, relate to the influence of the drug on the chemical reactions of various organic and inorganic substances. By the aid of these analytical procedures the pharmacologist accumulates a fund of data, equipped with which he can observe and interpret understandingly the action of the drug on the intact human body and can suggest its rational use in disease. Such methods as these have now been applied with more or less completeness toward the perfecting of a knowledge of the action of the older drugs, and no one of the newer remedies is employed without similar careful, preliminary experimental studies. The practical result is a vigorous reform of drug treatment. Physicians no longer administer the old mixtures of innumerable drugs, given with the comprehensive hope that some one component would hit the mark, and hence called "shot-gun" prescriptions. Large quantities of individual drugs also are avoided, and the endeavor is made to reach only the specific functions that are disordered.

Drugs affect living substance in one of two ways: either by increasing or by diminishing its natural activities. Thus, digitalis stimulates to greater contraction the muscle tissue in the walls of the arteries, and thus increases the blood pressure — at least in animals. Amyl nitrite, on the other hand, depresses these muscles and diminishes the blood pressure. In medicinal doses digitalis makes the heart beat more slowly, but it does this, not by depressing the heart muscle, but rather by stimulating the nervous mechanism whose normal action is to slow the heart. Atropin, however, an active principle of belladonna, quickens the heart by lessening the activity of the same nervous mechanism. Many drugs at first stimulate and then depress.

Drugs rarely affect similarly all the various kinds of cells in a body or indeed all the functions of the same cell. Thus strychnine seems to have a special predilection for the spinal cord and medulla oblongata, and within those parts it probably acts upon the incoming nervous paths rather than the outgoing. Quinine, on the contrary, seems to have no such choice, but affects nearly alike all kinds of the body's protoplasm. These selective peculiarities of drugs are a great aid to the physician, for they often enable him to reach a desired tissue with great exactness and without interfering with other tissues. They have never been so clearly demonstrated as in certain of the infectious diseases, *i.e.* diseases in which the causative agent is a specific living organism, such as a bacterium or a protozoan, which has invaded the body. It is obvious that in such a case the ideal drug would be one that would kill the parasites without injuring the patient. In several cases such drugs have been found. Quinine is such a specific for malarial germs. A compound of arsenic, atoxyl, has been found to be partially effective with the deadly African scourge, sleeping sickness; and still more effective bids fair to be a derivative of atoxyl, called arseno-phenyl-glycin. The most recent triumph of this nature is in the treatment of syphilis, which has been announced within a few months. This loathsome disease, the ultimate fate of the personally immoral, and terrible in its physical effects, dates from prehistoric times, and is perhaps the most widely distributed of all the major diseases. It is due to the ravages of a microscopic organism called *Treponema pallidum*, which possesses some of the characteristics of both bacteria and protozoa. Its body consists of a single cell, spiral in shape. It occurs within the tissues and within the blood of the infected human body. A few years ago Professor Paul Ehrlich, the director of the Royal Institute for Experimental Therapeutics at Frankfurt-on-the-Main, who has made very brilliant discoveries of value in both theoretical and practical pathology, began a search for a drug which should prove to be a specific for this organism. After investigating more than six hundred substances he found that the six hundred and sixth, a peculiar compound of arsenic, possesses, in many cases, the desired properties, namely, that of seeking out each and every *Treponema* in the body of the afflicted person and destroying it without injuring in any manner the body cells. Although the drug is not effective in every instance, it frequently happens that a single dose accomplishes the desired result. The popular name of this drug is 606, its medical name salvarsan, its chemical name dioxy-diamidoarseno-benzol. Ehrlich's work is prophetic of still greater possibilities, for if specific poisons have thus been discovered for two or three disease germs, we may confidently look for similar modes of treatment for others. It is possible that such specific chemicals will prove to be the medium of our final salvation from the infectious diseases.

Even when all the body cells are ultimately affected by a drug, it usually happens that some cells are more susceptible to it than others. This makes possible the practice of anesthesia. An anesthetic, like ether or chloroform, is a depressant of living substance : when its administration is continued, it diminishes and may ultimately put a stop to vital action and cause death. It acts upon all kinds of protoplasm and all varieties of cells and tissues, but in the early stages of its administration its action is more obvious upon the brain than upon other parts. Within the brain it depresses first those cells whose activities are accompanied by consciousness and therefore by the recognition of pain. Next in order of paralysis comes the spinal cord, which contains the central nervous mechanism of most of our bodily movements. And lastly comes the medulla oblongata, in which lies, among other important nervous centers, that center which maintains respiration. The successful administration of an anesthetic for a surgical operation demands that just so much of the drug be given as is required by the brain cells and the cells of the spinal cord to banish consciousness and the power of making bodily movements. With any amount beyond this, anesthesia approaches the danger point of stopping the breathing or the heart.

Much attention is now being given to the problem as to how drugs exert their action. How do they stimulate or depress protoplasm ? This problem is a difficult one, and its solution has hardly gone beyond the stage of hypothesis. It seems probable, however, that in many cases of drug action, if not in most, there is a chemical union between the drug and certain constituents of the cells. In some cases we can probably go even farther than this and link the reaction with specific parts of the molecules, or with the ions of the substances in question, or with the arrangement of the atoms within the molecule. If chemical union does occur, a selective action of a particular drug for a particular group of cells may be readily explained by supposing that such cells, and not others, contain particular chemical substances for which the drug has an affinity. In other cases the action of the drug is rather physical than chemical. Thus the subnitrate of bismuth, when taken into the stomach, forms an insoluble lining and thus protects the gastric walls from injurious agencies.

The ultimate fate of a drug varies with the variety of drug. Some drugs, for example, adrenalin, are actually destroyed by the tissues. Others are eliminated by the excretory organs, such as the kidneys, though in some cases this process is very slow. Thus, after a course of treatment with mercury the drug may be found in the body for two or three months.

A special division of drug therapy which has arisen in very recent years is that in which animal organs or preparations from such organs are administered in cases in which the analogous organs in men are wanting, are insufficiently developed or are diseased. In all of these cases the organs in question supply to the body an internal secretion which exercises a profound action on bodily metabolism, and the absence of which is followed by equally profound phenomena. So far the greatest success has attended such use of the thyroid glands in myxedema and cretinism. The many claims that have been made of the benefits following the administration of material from other organs must, at present, be received with caution.

Notwithstanding the many and varied improvements in drug therapy in recent years, it is undoubtedly a fact that with the development of other methods of dealing with disease, physicians are depending less than formerly on the conventional drugs. But there is truth in the words of the French clinician, "Medicine sometimes cures, it often relieves, it always consoles," and it will always continue to be used for all of these three purposes.

High hopes have been raised in the minds of some men of medicine that the newly discovered rays of various kinds will prove valuable in the treatment of disease. Roentgen rays and the emanations of radium have been turned to with the enthusiasm of expectant success. The physiological actions of these two agents are practically identical and vary with the intensity of the radiations. When they are weak they stimulate, when stronger they depress and may kill the living cells. Diseased tissue and pathological growths, such as tumors, seem to be more sensitive to the radiations than normal tissue. Sometimes the physician makes use of the stimulating action, and sometimes, as in tumors, the destructive action. The intensity of the dose of radiations should be carefully graded in accordance with the end desired and the variety of tissue dealt with. The selective action of the radiations on the different tissues is now becoming known, and the destructive burning which occurred with the early use of these agents can now usually be avoided. X-rays have been extensively used in diseases of the skin, and by both X-rays and radium certain tumors have undoubtedly been cured.   In a few other diseases specific symptoms have often been alleviated, but the limits of radiotherapy in general are not yet determined.

The therapeutic benefits resulting from proper bathing are now being emphasized more than ever before.   These consist not merely in the cleansing of the skin, for that is presupposed ; nor in the employment of medicated waters, for the absorption of such medicaments through the skin in such conditions does not occur ; but largely in the fact that water is a most suitable medium for conveying heat, cold, and mechanical stimuli to the sensory nerve-endings in the skin.   Afferent nervous impulses are thus produced, which in turn lead to beneficial reflex effects throughout the body, on the heart, the arteries, the respiratory organs, the nutritive processes, the bodily temperature, the distribution of blood corpuscles, the muscles, and the nervous system.   When properly regulated these actions may be turned to excellent account in the treatment of various diseases.   The cold bath employed in typhoid fever is valuable, less for any direct effect it may have in lowering the temperature, for this is slight, than for its reflex stimulating action on the bodily tissues.

Time forbids a consideration of the many other physical and chemical means of which the physician makes curative use, but we may turn to a method of healing of a different type which is of late attracting much attention, both popularly and among a considerable number of men of medicine, namely, mental healing or psychotherapy.   In all ages, from the most remote to the present, a close relation between mind and disease has been recognized.   This relation is not limited to the so-called diseases of the mind, but is conceded to exist for the great mass of both structural and functional diseases. In harmony with this belief the mind of the patient has always been one of the channels through which cure has been sought. Of late years, following the application of the experimental method to the study of mind, where introspection and metaphysical reasoning had long ruled, there is a tendency to introduce psychological principles into orthodox medicine. This has been more pronounced in France and Germany than in England and America, but the tendency is probably spreading. Outside of strictly medical circles there have arisen the cult of Christian Science and many less pretentious groups of healers, with all of whom treatment is based primarily upon psychic influences; and very recently certain long-established branches of the Christian church have come to believe that there exists for them a legitimate sphere of usefulness in the treatment of the sick.

That physical ills are responsible for mental changes, that the body can influence the mind, is a proposition which no one who has ever experienced physical ills will be disposed to deny. The psychic effect of pain, the hallucinations of fever, the cheerful hopefulness of tuberculosis, — all are well known. One's whole mental make-up may be profoundly affected by disease. "The devil when sick, the devil a monk would be."

But the truth of the reverse proposition, that the mind can influence the body and directly cure physical maladies, is not so evident. That there is a close relation between psychic states and the activity of parts of the body outside of the central nervous system, has been proved in many ways. Darwin published a volume on the external expression of the emotions in man and animals. Pawlow has found in animals that both the quantity and the composition of the saliva vary, not only in accordance with the presence of different kinds of food in the mouth, but with the mere exhibition of such foods, or even with the exhibition of geometrical forms or with musical sounds which have become associated with particular foods.   The watering of the mouth in the presence of delectable foods is thus literally true.   Cannon, by an ingenious use of X-rays, has made in animals a careful study of the movements occurring in the walls of the stomach and intestine during digestion, and has found that emotions, such as fear, distress, and rage, may be accompanied by a total cessation of the movements.   Peterson has demonstrated a close relation between emotions and electrical currents in the hands.   Mosso constructed a delicate balance, on the beam of which a man can lie horizontally.   If he is spoken to, the head end of the beam will immediately decline, owing to the passage of blood from his body to his brain.   The same change even follows a slight noise occurring during sleep. Because of the demand of the brain for blood, all sorts of mental processes are accompanied by a diminution of the volume of various parts of the body, such as the arm and the ear.   But none of these instances of close relationship between mental and corporeal processes demands, by way of explanation, that mind is responsible for bodily actions.

An unprejudiced reader of the mass of literature that has been poured upon a patient world concerning the relations of body and mind, cannot fail, if he has a sense of humor, to be impressed by its real grotesqueness in the midst of its seriousness.   A theory is elaborated with great completeness and subtlety of reasoning by one whom we will call philosopher A, and is proposed with a degree of conviction that would seem to win all.   Thereupon the equally acute philosopher B proceeds to show by the force of the abundant logic at his command that nothing is further from the truth than A's idea, that it is crude and inconceivable and inconsistent with known facts, and that B's conception is the only possible one. Then C enters the arena, and before the brilliance and strength of his arguments, not only does A go down, but B as well. C's hypothesis stands forth victorious, until it, too, is vanquished by the specious dialectician D. Thus we are asked to believe that both body and mind are material, and that they are both immaterial; that body is the product of mind, and mind the product of body; that body acts upon mind, that mind acts upon body, and that neither acts upon the other; that mind has no extension in space, and that it extends as far as thought extends. In such a state of divergence of opinions it would seem that a simple pragmatic position is justified, that any theory of the relations of body and mind that proves workable for the individual is in so far true.

Most physicians of the present time do not incline toward dialectic subtleties and do not formulate very exact theories of the relation of body and mind. In so far as they do so, probably many would incline toward some such notion as was outlined in my first lecture as a convenient working hypothesis for the physiologist.[1] All cells of the brain, as of other organs, manifest their activity by certain chemical and physical changes: they produce carbon dioxide and other substances, they become warmer, and they are the seat of electrical phenomena. Certain nerve-cells, such as those situated in the cortex of the cerebrum of the brain, manifest their activity, not only by the customary chemical and physical changes, but by certain other changes of an unknown nature, which we call psychic. Mind is the sum of these psychic phenomena. Differences in the activ-

[1] See p. 18.

ities of the cortical cells, resulting from corporeal changes, may be accompanied by differences in the chemical, physical, and psychical manifestations of these cells — in other words, body or brain may influence mind.   But, just as the carbon dioxide, heat, and electricity are the resultants, not the causes, of the activity of the brain cells, so is the psychic change a resultant and not a cause — in other words, mind cannot influence brain or body.   Every action of our nervous system may be likened to a link in a chain of neural or physiological processes, which is much branched and ever extending.   No one of the innumerable links ever arises *de novo;* it is always preceded by a past link.   It may or may not be followed by a future one : the ends of the chain's spreading branches may be linked to others or may terminate abruptly. But from the beginning of the individual's life to the end of it the chain itself is never broken.   Day and night, summer and winter, in season and out of season, our nervous tissues are ever active, and there is ever continuity.   Such continuity is one of causality; that is, each link is the resultant of those which have preceded it.   Most of our neural links are totally unconscious processes, but a few of them during our working hours exhibit the peculiarity which we call mind. Mind is one of the products of neural activity.   It is a psychic accompaniment of certain links in a continuous neural chain of cause and effect.   Mind is not necessarily continuous, and it is never causal in the sense that one idea can give rise to the next.   Such an hypothesis assumes nothing as to the nature of mind.   It leaves that for future investigation.   "But," an unbelieving critic would say, "your hypothesis would make forever impossible the use of mind as a therapeutic agent." That would seem to be literally true, and yet the methods employed by psychotherapists would still be justified.   Many of their cures are undoubted. It is only the interpretation of their cures that would be affected. Psychotherapy would still remain a legitimate agent to be employed by the physician.

In the present stage of the development of psychotherapy one cannot say in how far it will ultimately be used. Most physicians would probably restrict it to a limited range of nervous diseases, the exact anatomical basis of which is unknown. It is generally acknowledged to be of value in a class of diseases to which the general name psychoneuroses has been given. These include neurasthenia, psychasthenia, hysteria, and certain conditions bordering on insanity. But these names cover a wide range of disorders associated with organs outside of the central nervous system. Thus neurasthenia, which is only the modern, new-fangled name for the old malady nervous prostration, may be manifested by muscular weakness, various forms of indigestion, palpitation of the heart, and other disorders of the circulatory functions, deficiency of the various secreted fluids, a great variety of unwonted sensations, such as headache, backache, heat, cold, fatigue, soreness, numbness, weakness, various disturbances of vision, hearing, smell, and taste, abnormal mental phenomena and insomnia. Hysteria is a very complex disorder. Like neurasthenia, it may affect many bodily functions. It is specially characterized mentally by a lack of sensations of particular parts of the body, and by weakness of memory and the will. Psychasthenia is characterized preëminently by the presence of fixed ideas, or obsessions. Thus one patient had for years a morbid fear of dust in her room, and would sweep and dust and clean until she became exhausted. Later she devoted hours to the repeated washing of her hands. Here, too, are placed certain fears which many of us possess in a very mild form — fears of high places, of open places, or of closed rooms. In such states as these, all of which exhibit pronounced mental peculiarities, psychotherapy in the hands of intelligent, patient, and skillful physicians is frequently of great value.

Psychotherapeutic methods vary greatly with the individual physician, and there are many grades of complexity in treatment, from that involved in the simple, quiet reassuring manner of the old family doctor, to the long-continued, avowedly psychological treatment, following elaborate psychological analyses. Occasionally hypnosis is employed, but this is usually not regarded as necessary. The main factor in the treatment is probably suggestion. Through it old, harmful neural complexes are torn to pieces, and new, healthful ones are formed. The patient is taught how to inhibit wrong impulses and actions, and how to encourage right ones. The advantage of hypnosis consists in increasing the suggestibility of the patient. Most psychotherapists assume the existence of an unconscious mental state, which they term the subconscious mind, and believe that it is through this medium that suggestion acts. To the physiologist the phrase "subconscious mind" is a contradiction in terms. He prefers to regard mind and consciousness as synonymous, and so-called subconscious phenomena, however complex they may be, as neural phenomena, the ordinary physiological or physico-chemical processes of nervous tissues, to which no psychic qualities are added.

Psychotherapy, though it is centuries old, and though worthy endeavors are now being made in its behalf, is still hardly out of its infancy, and its growth on a really scientific or rational basis demands a much fuller knowledge than we possess at present of the ways in which nervous tissue normally works. Until such a physiological basis is secured, psychotherapy will continue to attract the charlatan and the credulous, the one to prey upon the other. That "mystery will lead millions by the nose" has been abundantly demonstrated in this field of mental healing. Hard-headed, mature men, who are masters of material things, will here lay aside their forceful intellects and think to find relief from physical ills in the seductive conceptions of unknown psychic forces. So-called healers are ever ready to take advantage of this human weakness. Even the presence of the body of the patient is no longer demanded. It can go about its business, and all unbeknown will still yield to absent treatment. In the midst of human ignorance and credulity and all the vagaries and deceptions of mind cure, scientific medicine has before it a great task of education.

IV

FROM time immemorial human life has been cursed by the two great evils of war and pestilence. Working at times together, at times apart, there is no portion of the earth and no race of men that they have not devastated. The one has slain its thousands, the other its millions, and sorrow and misery have ever accompanied and followed them. Ages have come and gone, while through them all the clash of arms has sounded and murderous plagues have silently spread unchecked. Now in the morning of the twentieth century the moral nature of man has risen against the one of these evils, and all his science is invoked against the other; and there is ground for the great hope that when our century passes away, they also will pass, and man will be freed forever from two of his greatest burdens.

The scientific features of modern medicine are nowhere more graphically illustrated than in the conquest of the infectious diseases. Scarcely a half century has elapsed since the nature of these diseases first became known; for it was during our Civil War that Louis Pasteur's labors were rapidly approaching their goal, and it was in 1876 that Robert Koch, in a study of anthrax, or splenic fever, conclusively demonstrated for the first time that a specific bacterium is the causative agent of a specific human disease. During this half century a whole new science, that of bacteriology,

64

has come into being, and mankind has for the first time learned to know the real meaning of sanitation.

The term "infectious disease" is applied to all those forms of disease which result from the invasion of the body by microscopic organisms. The micro-organisms, or germs, of most of the infectious diseases belong to the remarkable group of primitive creatures called bacteria. The authority of that ancient and unknown Hebrew, who once proclaimed that there is no thing new under the sun, received a rude shock toward the close of the seventeenth century, when Anton van Leeuwenhoek of Delft, by means of his newly invented glass lenses, showed to his fellow countrymen an unsuspected world of animalculæ in the midst of reputed Dutch cleanliness. The Jesuit priest, Kircher, is said to have been the first man to see bacteria, in 1659; but their importance in natural processes was not shown until one hundred and fifty years later, when Pasteur performed his immortal work. The successive steps of Pasteur's achievement are now well known — fermentation, spontaneous generation, the diseases of wines, the diseases of silkworms, the diseases of higher animals, and lastly hydrophobia. I trust that I will be pardoned if I here relate for the second time a personal experience concerning Pasteur.

In the summer of 1886 it was my good fortune to spend a few hours in the presence of this man in the rooms of the then newly organized Pasteur Institute in Paris. It was in the early days of the practical application of the results of his long-continued, devoted experimentation regarding the cause and treatment of hydrophobia. In a large room there was gathered together a motley company of perhaps two hundred persons, most of whom had been bitten by rabid animals. Men, women, and children, from the aged to babes in the arms

F

of their mothers, richly dressed and poorly dressed, gentle folk and rude folk, the burgher and the peasant; from the boulevards and the slums of Paris, from the north, south, east, and west of France, from across the channel in England, from the forests and steppes of Russia, where rabid wolves menace, from more distant lands and even from across the seas — all had rushed impetuously from the scene of their wounding to this one laboratory to obtain relief before it was too late. All was done systematically and in order. The patients had previously been examined and classified, and each class passed for treatment into a small room at the side: first, the newcomers, whose treatment was just beginning; then, in regular order, those who were in successive stages of the cure; and, lastly, the healed, who were about to be happily discharged. The inoculations were performed by assistants. But Pasteur himself was carefully overseeing all things, now assuring himself that the solutions and the procedure were correct, now advising this patient, now encouraging that one, ever watchful and alert and sympathetic, with that earnest face of his keenly alive to the anxieties and sufferings of his patients, and especially pained by the tears of the little children, which he tried to check by filling their hands from a generous jar of bonbons. It was an inspiring and instructive scene, and I do not doubt that to Pasteur, with his impressionable nature, it was an abundant reward for years of hard labor, spent partly in his laboratory with test-tubes and microscopes, and partly in the halls of learned societies, combating the doubts of unbelievers and scoffers, and compelling the medical world to give up its unscientific traditions and accept what he knew to be the truth.

Bacteria are regarded as rather more plant-like than animal-like in nature, although at such a low stage of existence no very sharp line of distinction can be drawn between plants and animals. A body of a bacterium consists of a single cell possessing a very simple constitution — a bit of protoplasm, probably some chromatin representing a nucleus, perhaps a cell wall and capsule, and occasionally swimming organs in the form of delicate projecting filaments. The bodies of most bacteria have the form of a sphere, a straight rod, or a spiral rod, and we therefore recognize the three groups of the coccus, the bacillus, and the spirillum. There is much difference in size among even individuals of a single species. One of the smallest known species is the bacillus of influenza or grippe, which is about $\frac{1}{50000}$ of an inch in length; one of the largest is the spirillum of relapsing fever, which may reach a length of even $\frac{1}{800}$ of an inch. The bacillus of typhoid fever varies in length from $\frac{1}{25000}$ of an inch to three times that figure. Probably species exist which are too small to be recognized even by the aid of our most efficient microscopes. When surrounded by abundant food the life of a single bacterium is very short. It is born by the division of its parent's body; for a brief period it tarries in its world to take food, grow, and perform its good or evil work; and then its body is split into the bodies of its two offspring — and that is all the life and immortality it knows. The duration of the life of a single cholera germ under favorable conditions has been estimated at twenty minutes, and its possible descendants in one day at 1600 trillions. If the lot of the bacterium is not cast in pleasant places, and it faces a precarious existence, it may concentrate its substance, develop a resistant coat, and become an inactive and hardy spore. In this state it rests until its environment becomes again favorable for growth. Bacteria have the reputation of being very hardy creatures, but this is only partly justified by fact. Most species can survive a brief exposure to extreme cold, some species even so extreme a temperature as 300° F. below zero, and though prolonged cold may kill them, ice not infrequently contains living germs. Heat is more quickly fatal, and boiling water is sufficient to kill all microbes that are likely to be present in it. When in liquids, ten minutes' exposure to heat is fatal to typhoid bacilli at 133° F. Bacterial spores are much more resistant to heat, though it is gratifying to know that the formation of spores is not very common with those species that are responsible for diseases. Sunlight is very destructive to bacteria, but, unfortunately, they can readily penetrate to places to which the sun's rays can never hope to follow. Thorough drying is also destructive, and renders innocuous most germs within a few hours or a few days, although here also spores are more resistant. Many chemical substances are poisonous to bacteria; and valuable among these as disinfectants or germicides are formaldehyde, carbolic acid, bichloride of mercury, and sulphate of copper.

Between one thousand and fifteen hundred species of bacteria altogether have been described. It is probable that these species are constant and that one does not pass into another. Moreover, there is no evidence that new species are now arising. Bacteria may be distinguished from one another partly by their microscopic appearance, though thus only in a limited degree, but chiefly by other characters, such as the kind of food required by them, their manner of growth, their chemical reactions, their products, their relation to the factors of their environment, their behavior toward staining reagents, and other general biological activities. We ought to be very sparing of a general condemnation of bacteria. Most of the known species live outside of animal organisms, and many of these are of great importance to the welfare and pleasure of mankind. Of such as are beneficent to man I might mention those which perform many of the helpful fermentations and putrefactions of organic matter; those which replenish worn-out soils by abstracting nitrogen from the atmosphere and offering it in a form available for the growth of plants; those which ripen cream and thus transmit to butter its pleasant flavor; those which are engaged in the making of cheese; and those which tan hides and thus make leather possible. Certain souls may question the beneficence of certain other species which contribute to the pleasure of man. Among these I may mention those that aid in the curing of tobacco and those that contribute to the fermentation of wines. A certain number of bacteria have, in the course of time, come to be parasitic upon animals and men. Some of these are harmless, some are probably beneficial, and a few are the producers of disease. We know nothing of the way in which bacteria came to reside in the human body. Medicine has no Milton to tell of this in stately verse. But if the fall of man really "Brought death into the world and all our woe," perhaps the fatal apple was the bearer of man's first disease germs.

The paths by which bacteria enter the body are comparatively few. A healthy uninjured skin forms a coat of armor that is practically impenetrable by them, except when they are brought by intermediate hosts, such as biting insects. But our bodies must have inlets and outlets, and these, together with skin wounds, are the danger points. If we breathe — and we must breathe — floating germs may come to our air passages and lungs. If we eat or drink — and we must eat and drink — germs may enter our mouths and may pass on to our stomachs and intestines. Doubtless the danger of infection from breathing is popularly exaggerated, and in general is not so great as the danger from whatever is placed in the mouth. Bacteria are very light and can float in air for a considerable time, but though the air is one considerable source of tuberculosis and probably of influenza, most floating bacteria are probably either dead or not pathogenic. To the mouth go water, milk, uncooked food, unclean dishes, hands, and other objects, all of which may be the carriers of pathogenic germs.

While the entrance of bacteria into the body should, if possible, be prevented, it is gratifying to know that the presence there, even of pathogenic species, does not ensure diseases. Doubtless all of us at this moment are carrying, each within his own person, the living germs of pneumonia and various minor ailments, while some of us probably possess the bacilli of tuberculosis, influenza, and perhaps diphtheria. But this, however, need give us no alarm. One swallow cannot make a summer, nor can one germ make a disease, except in the rarest of cases. Usually many of the same kind are required. Moreover, the individual bacteria of a species vary in virulence, a property that is not well understood; and a certain degree of virulence is required if the disease is to appear. There are many close analogies in behavior between the seeds of a higher plant sown in the ground, and the germs of a disease planted in the human body. The sower who went forth to sow found that, what with the fowls of the air, the stones of the earth, the heat of the sun, and the thorns, only that seed which fell on good ground brought forth fruit. So bacteria, after entering a body, find many trials awaiting them: the body may possess an immunity against them ; there is no soil in which they can thrive ; and they have enemies to overcome. Some of these difficulties are now understood, while some are still mysterious.

In the preceding lecture I spoke of some of the natural defenses of the body against disease.[1] I wish now to amplify this subject with reference to bacteria. If the latter enter the air passages of the nose, pharynx, trachea, or lungs, they are very liable to become caught in the mucus that is secreted by the cells in the walls of these passages, and to be swept outward again by the innumerable cilia which are restlessly sweeping the surfaces. Some of them may, however, find lodgment on the mucous membranes. Many of those which reach the stomach are killed by its acid and are digested by the gastric juice. Some, however, such as cholera and typhoid germs, if they succeed in passing the stomach, find a more congenial environment in the intestine. If in the mucous membranes of the air passages and the alimentary canal there chance to be places where, because either of mechanical injury or nutritional disturbance, the tissues do not possess their usual degree of healthy resisting power, the bacteria may find the breaches in the walls and push their way in, just as they may also enter through wounds in the skin. Once within the tissues, some varieties, like the germs of diphtheria and tetanus, found colonies at their place of entrance; others are carried by the blood to more satisfactory local regions; while still others do not remain in one locality, but continue to share the rushing, changing life of the constantly moving blood. Wherever they chance to abide, if they find food, an agreeable temperature, and other satisfactory conditions of life, they proceed to grow and multiply. Then begins a struggle for supremacy between the established and organized tissues of the body and the unorganized horde of invaders. To learn the intricate details of this struggle has required the labors of an army of investigators, many of

[1] See p. 42.

them leaders in scientific medicine. Fact has led to hypothesis, hypothesis to further fact; theories have been proposed and discarded; and gradually, out of the complex maze, there has arisen a great body of truth. Though the labor is incomplete as yet, and its end is probably still far away, it is interesting, both as an example of remarkable scientific achievement and as affording a basis not only for an immediate saving of many lives, but also for an ultimately complete conquest of the infectious diseases.

Bacteria sometimes interfere with bodily processes in a merely mechanical way, as any other foreign matter in large quantity within the tissues might interfere. But they are chiefly harmful through peculiar chemical substances which they produce. These substances are poisonous or toxic to living substance, and are hence called toxins. Some of them are powerful poisons: the toxin of tetanus is said to be about two hundred times more poisonous than strychnine. The toxins appear to be of two kinds. One kind, the exotoxins, are freely given out during the life of the bacterial cell; the other, the endotoxins, are locked tightly within the cell and are only released at its death and dissolution. The relative quantities of these two vary with the varieties of bacteria: the poisonous properties of the germs of diphtheria and tetanus are due preëminently to their exotoxins; those of cholera, typhoid fever, and pneumonia to their endotoxins. Once the toxins are set free, they are carried by the blood to all parts of the body, and they may be absorbed by the body cells and exert their poisonous action. They constitute the more immediate cause of the disease. An infectious disease, therefore, is substantially a poisoning of the body by a powerful chemical substance. The common symptoms of such a disease are fever, chills, a rapid pulse, headache, delirium, muscular weakness, general prostration, and often characteristic rashes or eruptions in the skin. A certain period must always elapse between the advent of the bacteria and the appearance of the symptoms in sufficient force to indicate the presence of the disease. During this period of incubation the bacteria are growing and multiplying and producing their toxins. The period of incubation of most infectious diseases is less than one week, of typhoid fever usually from eight to fourteen days. When unopposed and not terminating fatally, the disease usually runs a definite course, becoming at first for a time more and more severe, then reaching its culmination, and finally slowly abating.

But the body does not passively submit to the ravages of its unwelcome invaders. It has many means of defense, and these are automatically put into action as soon as the enemy appears. The two obviously direct ways of dealing with the situation would appear to be, first, to prevent existing toxins from exerting their deleterious action, and, secondly, to destroy the bacteria and thus prevent the formation of more toxins. The body, of its own accord, makes use of both of these methods. It opposes at least the exotoxins with antitoxins, and it opposes bacteria with antibacterial agencies and leucocytes. It is worth our while to consider these methods of defense more fully.

It has been found that whenever foreign matter, such as living or dead organisms or the products of organisms, is introduced into the tissues of an animal, the animal's cells are stimulated to produce chemical substances which are in certain ways antagonistic to the foreign matter, and tend to protect the animal's body from it. To these protective substances the general name antibodies has been given. Many varieties of antibodies have already been recognized, and undoubtedly others exist, as yet unknown. Antitoxins constitute one group of antibodies. When a specific toxin attacks the living cells of an individual body, the cells may ultimately succumb, but this may not occur until they have made efforts to resist the attack. They are stimulated by the toxin to manufacture a specific substance, the antitoxin, which has an affinity for the corresponding toxin and the power of neutralizing its poison. They manufacture this in considerable quantities, much more than is required for neutralizing the small amount of toxin that attacks the cells in question, and the excess is generously poured out of the cell, circulates through the body with the lymph or blood, and may unite with whatever free toxin it chances to meet. This marriage of toxin and antitox·n renders the toxin harmless, and thus other cells are protected.

While some of the body cells are thus busy in the formation of antitoxin, either the same cells or others engage in another kind of protective labor by the production of antibodies which are destructive to the bacteria. These have been called antibacterial, bactericidal, or bacteriolytic substances, or, in brief, bacteriolysins. There are different theories regarding the process by which bacteria are destroyed, but there is general agreement in the fact that two antibodies are engaged in it. One of these is the actual destructive agent, but it can act only with the coöperation of the other. If we accept a very helpful conception of Ehrlich, we must believe that there is normally present within the blood a quantity of the destructive agent, which he calls complement, while the coöperative agent, which he calls immune body or amboceptor, is produced by the body cells when stimulated by the bacteria. The amboceptor acts as a middleman between the complement and the bacterium, bringing about the chemical union of the two. This union is fatal to the bacterial cell, for after taking its complement it becomes quiet and its substance breaks up into granules and gradually dissolves — and thus the unwelcome guest is disposed of.

With some diseases, however, there is a certain degree of danger to the body involved in a wholesale destruction of the bacteria contained within it. These are the diseases of which the bacterial poisons are endotoxins. These toxins differ from other bacterial toxins in that they are locked within the living substance of the bacterial cells, and are freed only on the death of the latter. The relations of endotoxins are not yet altogether elucidated. The body cells do not seem to be capable of manufacturing antitoxins for them, and we do not know definitely how the body defends itself against them, but it seems that if a large quantity of them are rapidly set free, they may poison the tissues and cause death. They afford a further instance of the varied agencies by which bacteria may overcome the body.

Investigators have discovered many other antibodies besides antitoxins and antibacterial substances, which are capable of exerting still other actions; but their significance in the subject under discussion, namely, the mutual relations of bacteria and the body, is not yet altogether clear. One fact of great interest, however, is that antibodies are among the most highly specialized substances of which we have knowledge. Each is adapted to the special work for which it was created, and to no other. The antitoxin of diphtheria cannot neutralize the toxin of tuberculosis. The antibacterial substance that is destructive to diphtheria germs is ineffective with the germs of tuberculosis or typhoid or erysipelas or pneumonia. As Ehrlich has expressed it: "Antitoxins and antibacterial substances are, so to speak, charmed bullets, which strike only those objects for whose destruction they have been produced by the organism." Hence if two varieties of bacteria happen to attack the body at the same time, each comes into conflict with the weapons best adapted to cope with its own peculiar means of warfare. The ingenuity of the body in meeting the exact conditions presented to it seems to be almost without limit.

Ehrlich, who has been one of the most stimulating and suggestive investigators of the antibodies, has proposed a very helpful scheme for interpreting the mutual relations of bacteria and the body cells, and has pictured it in graphic form. Both his conception and his figures have been very helpful in enabling us to understand what are, in reality, very complex processes. He believes these relations to be analogous to those that hold between food and the body cells. From the standpoint of nutrition, he considers it possible to classify the chemical substances of which the cell is composed into two main groups of substances, distinguished by the respective duties which they have to perform. There is the main mass of cell substance which carries on the special activities that characterize the cell; and then there are special clusters of atoms whose duty it is to bring this main mass into relations with the varied substances in the environment. These clusters of atoms, which may be very numerous, may be appropriately called receptors, and it is only through its receptors that the cell is able to take food and other matter. Each receptor is adapted to receive only its appropriate material — one receptor one kind of food or other matter, another receptor another kind. Some receptors are adapted to receive the toxins of particular species of bacteria; others are adapted to the bacteria themselves. If a toxin happens along and meets its appropriate receptor, a chemical union between the two takes place. The toxin may kill the cell, or it may stimulate the cell to produce and set free other similar receptors. These free receptors constitute the antitoxin. Or a bacterium may happen along and find its appropriate receptor, and again a union takes place; again the cell is stimulated, and its amboceptors are set free.

But the story of the struggle between bacteria and the body is not yet complete. In some way not fully understood the presence of bacteria arouses to action certain varieties of the white corpuscles of the blood. Isolated bacteria may be attacked by isolated leucocytes; and a localized crowd of bacteria may become the center of a crowd of leucocytes. The latter proceed to fall upon the invaders and devour and digest them. This process is known as phagocytosis, and for the time the hungry leucocytes are phagocytes. Metchnikoff was the first man to make known the phagocytic activities of the white blood corpuscles, and has constantly insisted upon their great importance in combating bacterial diseases.[1] Quite recently Sir Almroth Wright, of London, and others have extended our knowledge. It had been known for some time that the extent to which phagocytosis occurs in a given body differs greatly at different times. Sometimes the leucocytes will take in no bacteria at all, or only a few; sometimes they will take in many; sometimes they will cram themselves so full as almost to burst. It was suspected that these differences in behavior were due to some unknown substance in the blood, and it was thought at first that this substance stimulated the leucocytes and made them eager for bacterial food. But later it was concluded from experiments on rabbits that the substance must act on the bacteria themselves, rather than the leucocytes; and about

[1] See also p. 45.

six years ago this became clear. The unknown substance has now been shown to constitute a class of antibodies, to which the name opsonins has been given, from the Greek word meaning "to prepare food for." Opsonins exist more or less abundantly in the blood and among the tissues. They are absorbed by the bacteria and affect them in such a manner as to render them palatable to the leucocytes, who are irresistibly drawn toward the bacteria and surround, engulf, kill, and digest them. Opsonins are just now receiving much attention from scientific investigators. Their origin is not yet clear — they are probably manufactured and given off to the blood plasma by the leucocytes. Their relation to other antibodies is not altogether understood — it has been suggested that they are identical with some of the antibacterial substances. They seem to be always present in the body, though their quantity varies greatly. There seem to be many varieties of them, and each variety is adapted to one kind of bacterium : typhoid opsonins are taken up by typhoid bacilli; pneumonia opsonins by pneumococci. The degree to which the germs of any disease are destroyed by leucocytes depends on the quantity of the specific opsonin that is present. If there is an abundance of it, phagocytosis becomes a most valuable aid in ridding the body of bacteria.

Thus the body's methods of defense against its hostile immigrants are three in number. It neutralizes the bacterial toxins by antitoxins; it destroys bacteria by antibacterial substances; and it also destroys bacteria by its phagocytes with the aid of opsonins. It does not appear, however, to employ all of these methods to an equal degree with any one disease. Thus in diphtheria both antitoxin and phagocytes are important, but the destruction of the germs by antibacterial substances seems to be very doubtful. In cholera the antibacterial method is perhaps the sole one employed. In typhoid and pneumonia phagocytosis is probably the chief method, while in dysentery and the plague antibacterial substances seem to play the principal rôle. We do not know how there happen to be these differences, and there is still much divergence of opinion concerning the actual mode of defense in different cases. Of the three methods it seems at present probable that the most nearly universal one is phagocytosis. The simple, little, wandering, primitive, white blood cells appear to be our chief protectors against bacterial enemies. They are our soldiers, our national guardsmen, our policemen all together; and, if the world ever chooses to bestow honor upon any single part, instead of the whole of a man, its chiefest homage ought to be paid to these lowliest of cells.

Bacteria are not the only variety of microscopic beings that bring disease to man. From what we know of them it is not surprising to learn that other forms of low organisms have acquired a similar parasitic habit of living, and that man is made to suffer from these also. These other organisms to which I refer belong to the lowest order of animal life, the protozoa. Although their bodies consist of but a single cell, protozoa both structurally and functionally, stand higher in the biological scale of organisms than do bacteria. Their protoplasm often includes more or less elaborate structures, such as mineral substance serving as a skeleton, primitive muscle, cilia for locomotion and the capture of food, a mouth and a primitive œsophagus, contractile vacuoles, which serve as primitive excretory organs, and a double nucleus. Various physiological functions are often highly developed in them, examples of which are the power to respond to stimuli, the coordination of different parts of their cell, and various metabolic activities. They reproduce by both asexual and sexual processes. The group of the protozoa is a very large one, and, although the number of species that are parasitic in man's body is considerable, those that have been conclusively recognized as the causative agents in human diseases are scarcely more than four or five. These diseases comprise malaria, the sleeping sickness of Africa, and the tropical fevers which have been variously named, such as dumdum fever, and kala azar. In these cases the germs have a somewhat elaborate life history, with two stages, which are passed respectively in the bodies of human beings and certain species of insects. Human beings receive the germs through the bites of infected insects, and thus infected, they may also transmit the germs if they are bitten by other insects. The life history of the malarial organism is best known, having been very fully worked out about ten years ago. At least three species, if not four, of simple protozoa have been recognized as the germs of the various types of malarial disease. Within the infected human body they live in the red corpuscles of the blood. They multiply asexually, and destroy the corpuscles. While man is thus one of their hosts, the mosquito of the genus *Anopheles* is the other. Why nature should have ordained that only the female mosquito shall suck the blood of its victim, and hence be the sole carrier of the germs, is not clear. Yet such is the fact. Within the stomach of the insect the germs thrive and multiply sexually, and ultimately they swarm through the body and reach the salivary gland. Here they await their transmission to the body of the next human victim, and thus the cycle is continued.

The relation of the protozoan *Trypanosoma* to the deadly African sleeping sickness has been demonstrated within ten years. The organism is a long cell, twisted somewhat spirally, and is continually moving by means of a delicate undulating membrane attached along one edge and extended at the posterior end into a freely whipping flagellum. It is transmitted to its human victim by the bite of the tse-tse fly, *Glossina palpalis*. It lives at first within the blood, and later appears in the cerebro-spinal fluid. It multiplies actively, and produces fever, emaciation, somnolence, and ultimately coma and death. Its full life history is not known.

Almost nothing is known regarding the chemical or metabolic activities of the pathogenic protozoa and the reactions to them on the part of their hosts. Protozoan diseases, however, resemble in many ways bacterial diseases, and it is probable that the germs of the former also produce toxins and are opposed by antibodies, but here is an opportunity for research.

The infectious diseases, indeed, still offer abundant opportunities for investigation. For a considerable number of them there is yet no certainty as to the identity of the organism that causes them. There is a certain amount of evidence that protozoa are responsible for rabies, smallpox, scarlet fever, trachoma, and a form of dysentery called amebic dysentery. Thus, minute particles which suggest protozoan forms are found in the brain cells of victims of rabies, and in the skin cells of those of smallpox. But in all of these cases conclusive evidence as to the nature of the causative organisms is wanting. Mumps, measles, typhus fever, infantile paralysis, yellow fever, and some other undoubted infections still defy all search for the germinal agent. In the case of infantile paralysis and of yellow fever the virus retains its infectious property, even after being filtered through a fine porcelain filter. It is therefore suspected that the germs are too minute to be recognized with the present powers of our microscopes.

We who live our lives in civilized communities are subject to a malady, in itself not serious, which is the cause of great personal annoyance, is often the forerunner of dangerous disease, and contributes in many ways to man's misery. I refer to our common enemy, "colds." A "cold" is characterized by a congestion and swelling of the tissues forming the walls of the air passages of the nose and throat, a mucous secretion from the walls which is at first watery and irritating and later becomes thicker, soreness of the throat and pain in swallowing, hoarseness, sneezing and coughing, an abundant secretion of tears, headache, slight fever, a rapid pulse, a dry skin, an impairment of the senses of smell, taste, and hearing, and sometimes bronchial irritation. There may be an accumulation of pus in the middle ear and in the cavities of the frontal and cheek bones. The term "cold" is employed loosely and is a misnomer, since the malady does not necessarily have any relation to external cold. Different technical names are given to it in accordance with the locality in which the symptoms are most pronounced, and thus a "cold" may be a rhinitis, a pharyngitis, a laryngitis, or even a bronchitis. It is now generally acknowledged that, whatever its locality, it is caused by bacteria and is contagious. Various attempts have been made to discover its causative germ, and there are differences of opinion as to the latter's identity. Two organisms, called *Bacillus coryzæ segmentosus* and *Micrococcus catarrhalis*, have been found to be commonly and abundantly present in the air passages during acute attacks of "cold," and are believed by some investigators to be chiefly responsible for the common symptoms. Other bacteria, such as the pneumococcus, the pneumobacillus, the streptococcus, the staphylococcus, and the bacillus of influenza, are not infrequent. According to our present knowledge, therefore, a "cold" appears to be not a specific disease caused by a single species of organism, but rather an infection resulting from the activities of several species, some of which, at least, live constantly upon the surfaces of the air passages. We have little exact knowledge of the bodily conditions under which these organisms, some of which are harmless ordinarily, suddenly begin to thrive, multiply, and perform their offensive work. Exposure of the body to external cold and to drafts of air, which are popularly believed to be the chief causes of colds, is probably less potent than many other general conditions, such as fatigue, indigestion, and the maltreatment of the body in many ways.

It might here prove interesting to consider some of the specific media that have been demonstrated to convey disease germs to the human body. It is known that the bacilli of typhoid fever may be carried into the body in water, milk, oysters, and other solid food, and by means of infected fingers or articles of household use. Probably water and milk are the chief carriers of typhoid germs. They may be transmitted from the dejecta of human beings to these media in various ways, but it seems undoubted that house flies are not infrequent carriers of them. The germs of diphtheria have been proved to be disseminated in milk, but probably the most common media of their transmission are personal articles, such as clothing, toys, and common drinking cups. The germs of tetanus are received through wounds in the skin when they have become contaminated with soil, dust from various sources, particles from the explosive caps of toy pistols, rusty nails, and other articles on which the tetanus bacilli may survive. The germs of scarlet fever may be conveyed by infected milk and also by personal articles which have been in contact with those afflicted by the disease. The germs of tuberculosis may likewise be acquired by personal articles, by the breathing of germ-laden air, through the medium of milk, at least in children, and probably occasionally by means of butter and cheese. The germs of cholera are conveyed by water, milk, raw foods, such as salads, which have been washed in infected water, and by personal articles. House flies may carry them. Malaria and yellow fever result only from organisms conveyed by the bites of certain species of mosquitoes, which have become infected from other human beings. The bacilli of the plague are conveyed partly by human contact and personal effects, and partly by the bites of fleas which have become infected from rats and other animals. The germs of smallpox are transmitted by personal contact, and probably by the air. Hydrophobia results from organisms received from the bites of rabid animals which have been bitten by other rabid animals.

The more the dissemination of bacteria is studied, the clearer it appears that the most nearly universal mode of transmission of the more widely distributed infectious diseases is through contact with an infected person and infected personal articles. This view is supported by much evidence, drawn from the careful tracing of the sources of specific infections. It has also come to be recognized that many of those who carry the living germs do not at the time possess the disease, may never have possessed it in the past, nor are they destined necessarily to possess it in the future. Such persons have come to be known as bacteria carriers, and, although they appear to be in good health, they may be the unwitting transmitters of the disease to others. Bacteria carriers are undoubtedly active in the spread of diphtheria and typhoid fever, and probably of pneumonia, influenza, epidemic cerebro-spinal meningitis, infantile paralysis, and many other diseases. The germs of diphtheria, pneumonia, and influenza survive in the throat, those of epidemic meningitis and infantile paralysis in the nose, and those of typhoid fever in the gall bladder and the intestine. The case of "typhoid Mary" has become historic in the annals of New York medicine, the unfortunate woman whose trail as a domestic servant was marked by the frequent appearance of typhoid fever in the families of her employers. Twenty-six cases of the disease were thus traced to her as the source of infection. Several hundred cases were recently traced by Dr. Park of the Department of Health of the City of New York to the milk supplied from a farm employing a man who had had typhoid forty-seven years before. Many localized outbreaks of disease, which appear to be purely spontaneous and have no causal connection with other cases, are probably due to bacteria-carriers. It appears to be difficult to destroy the germs within the bodies of such individuals, who are often a serious menace to society. This recent discovery by scientific medicine thus presents a new sociological problem, the solution of which is not evident.

V

THE TREATMENT AND THE PREVENTION OF INFECTIOUS DISEASES

THE time-honored treatment by the physician of a patient suffering from a severe infectious disease has varied in detail from time to time, but has consisted in general of an alleviation of the various symptoms and a promotion of the individual's general well-being. If pain were present, it could be relieved by drugs. If there were fever, it could be diminished by drugs. If there were general prostration, rest and food would tend to counteract it. But no one of these measures touched the heart of the difficulty. Until very recently drugs had proved of specific curative value in but two instances: quinine in malaria and mercury in syphilis. It is true that, if given in quantity, other drugs would kill the germs, but such quantities as were required for this purpose would kill the patient as well, and however effective they might be with the disease, there were obvious objections to a course of treatment that would thus terminate. With the single exception of Jenner's discovery in 1796 of the value of vaccination in smallpox, it was not until the year 1885, scarcely twenty-five years ago, that more specific methods began to be employed to aid mankind in his struggle with infectious diseases. In that year Pasteur introduced his method of combating rabies. This was the beginning of a new era, and in the treatment and the prevention of the infectious diseases modern medicine has demonstrated most serviceable practical powers, and has won brilliant triumphs.

Scarcely a year now passes without some valuable addition to our resources in dealing with these greatest of mankind's bodily scourges. The new methods are possible partly because we have at last come to recognize the causative agents of many of these diseases, partly because we have discovered means of cultivating bacteria outside of living bodies, and partly because we can produce the diseases in the bodies of living animals and study their course and their treatment under conditions which we can control. Without this method of animal experimentation, indeed, our knowledge would be mainly of scientific interest.

Bacteriologists have shown great ingenuity in devising methods by which bacteria may be cultivated and studied. Their laboratories have become veritable bacteriological gardens, where living germs are kept under the very best possible conditions. The species are separated from one another; the proper foods are given to each; the most advantageous surroundings, as to light, temperature, air, and moisture, are provided; the bacteria are nursed when ill; and every effort is made that they may lead healthy lives. Opportunities are thus given for the exact study of their activities.

When, a quarter of a century ago, this study had given some notions of the life history of bacteria, it began to dawn upon investigators that, if they could provide the unfortunate person attacked by the germs with an additional supply of his own weapons, those substances which are antagonistic to the bacteria or bacterial toxins and are specifically fitted to meet their attacks, he would have greater resources with which to fight the disease. Antibodies are nature's own remedies, harmless to the patient, but fatal to the germs and an antidote to their poisons. The argument that because a thing is nature's own it must therefore be superior to a similar object of man's device is an argument that may easily be refuted by facts. Helmholtz is credited with saying that if an instrument-maker should send to him an optical apparatus as imperfect as the human eye, he would return it. The common version of the tale is probably an exaggeration. No one recognized more clearly than Helmholtz the marvelous powers and adaptability of the human eye, and yet, exact physicist as he was, he was acutely aware of the imperfections of the human lenses, imperfections that would not be tolerated in the optical instruments of the present time. Man cannot make a human eye, but he can make a lens that is largely free from chromatic and spherical aberration and astigmatism. In the treatment of the infectious diseases man has not yet discovered agencies that surpass or even approach those that nature herself has devised, unless the two or three examples of specific drugs be so considered, but he has been able to direct in certain ways nature's methods of obtaining and employing these agencies. When nature sets to work to prepare substances antagonistic to bacteria or their products, she introduces her bacteria into living bodies, and by them the body cells are stimulated to manufacture and pour out into the blood the desired antibodies. From man's standpoint it is a heroic method. It is the old struggle for existence, which nature is always fond of, and in which it is not foretold whether man or the microbe shall prove to be the fitter to survive. Now scientific medicine steps in, and tries to give man the advantage of its knowledge.

Two methods are now employed in the treatment of these diseases: one is to obtain from some source, other than the body of the patient, a quantity of the specific antibodies, and turn them over to him; the other is to give to him specific substances which can stimulate his own cells to be more active in the production of antibodies. These methods are called respectively the serum method and the vaccine method.

In the employment of the serum method a culture is made of the species of bacterium that is the causative agent in the disease. This should be a pure culture, free from contamination with other species. Either some of these bacteria or the toxins produced by them are injected into the body of a suitable animal. The animal's cells are thereby stimulated to produce antibodies, and cast them out into its blood. In some cases these antibodies are antitoxins; in other cases they are antibacterial substances, or opsonins. When the animal's blood has acquired a considerable quantity of them, it is drawn, and allowed to clot. From the more solid portion of the clot the serum or liquid part is then removed. It contains, dissolved within it, the antibodies. Serum in itself has no curative power; it is simply a medium of holding the antibodies, and is curative only in so far as it contains curative antibodies. When used it is injected into the patient's body, and thus he is given a large stock of defensive agencies at an earlier time than he is able to provide them unaided. Specific serums are useful in dealing with diseased conditions that have already made their appearance, but they may also profitably be given to an individual in whose body the bacteria either have not yet appeared or have not got a considerable foothold, and thus an attack of the disease may be forestalled. Their use as preventive agents, indeed, is often of greater value than their curative use. Serums have now been employed for a considerable number of infectious diseases. Some of them have proved their efficiency, and some have not.

Before considering them in further detail, I wish to say a

few words regarding the significance and proper mode of interpretation of medical statistics. The assertion that statistics may be made to prove anything is as frequent as the assurance that figures will not lie. The term " mortality," as applied to diseases, has two meanings : it may signify either the number of deaths in proportion to the population, or the number of deaths in proportion to the number of persons attacked by the disease. The former may be called the total mortality, or death rate, the latter the case mortality. The two do not necessarily vary *pari passu*. Thus, if an epidemic occurs and more persons are attacked by the disease than before, more may die and the total mortality may be higher. But if at the same time better methods of treatment are used, the percentage of attacked persons who die may be less than before, and thus, although total mortality may be higher, case mortality may be lower. In determining whether a certain method of treatment is efficacious or not within a limited period of time or a limited locality, it is obvious that the significant fact is the percentage of cures among those who have received the treatment, or the case mortality. Umbrellas will not prevent the rain from falling, but they may diminish the number of persons who get wet. In the long run, however, an efficient remedy for an infectious disease will gradually diminish the total death rate from the disease, and will tend to eliminate it wholly from the earth's surface. I speak of this matter of the significance of the term mortality, because it has happened that certain persons hostile to the new therapy have misinterpreted the statistics, either ignorantly or wilfully, and thus have attempted to justify their prejudices.

Diphtheria antitoxin began to be used experimentally in the year 1892, and within the subsequent three or four years it spread over the whole world.   It is produced by injecting into young, vigorous, healthy horses a powerful toxin obtained from a virulent culture of the bacillus of diphtheria.   Doses of the toxin, at first small and then gradually increasing in quantity, are injected hypodermically at intervals of from three to seven days.   Stimulated by this toxin, the horse's cells produce antitoxin, and at intervals the antitoxic strength of his blood is tested.   Usually after two or three months it is powerful enough for therapeutic use.   Blood is then drawn from the animal's jugular vein, with little inconvenience to himself, at intervals of perhaps one week for several months, regular injections of toxin still being continued.   The antitoxic strength of the blood usually diminishes in the course of time, and the animal is then allowed a period of freedom from inoculation.   Later it may be resumed, and a suitable horse may thus periodically furnish strong serum for several years. The blood after withdrawal is allowed to coagulate and the serum loaded with antitoxin oozes from the clot, is drawn off with strict aseptic precautions, and is placed in suitable bottles.   Sometimes a small quantity of an antiseptic is added to it, although if kept in a cool dark place it remains in good condition during many months without antiseptic treatment ; in time it undergoes a slow deterioration.   Dr. Park and his staff of the Department of Health of the City of New York have devised methods by which the antitoxin may be freed from most of the other constituents of the serum, and thus may be obtained in concentrated form.   Its amount in the serum may be determined by testing its protecting power on guinea pigs which have been inoculated with a standard toxin.   The unit of antitoxin is that amount that will neutralize one hundred minimal fatal doses of such a standard toxin.   The antitoxin is always thus standardized at the laboratories before it is allowed to be used. When employed with human beings it is injected either subcutaneously or directly into a vein, the latter being the more quickly effective method of administration and advisable in serious cases. For the prevention of diphtheria from 300 to 1000 units may be employed, and for treatment after the disease has appeared, from 1500 to 20,000 units.

DEATHS FROM DIPHTHERIA AND CROUP IN THE BOROUGHS OF MAN-
HATTAN AND THE BRONX, CITY OF NEW YORK

YEAR	NUMBER OF DEATHS PER 100,000 OF POPULATION	CASE MORTALITY IN PERCENTAGE
1888	167.7	39.3
1889	146.2	35.3
1890	110.5	38.7
1891	118.7	36.7
1892	123.3	40.6
1893	145.5	36.2
1894	158.6	29.7
1895 Antitoxin came into general use .	105.5	18.8
1896	92.5	15.4
1897	81.9	14.6
1898	46.7	12.1
1899	53.8	13.2
1900	62.0	15.2
1901	57.9	15.9
1902	52.3	10.9
1903	54.7	10.6
1904	54.8	10.4
1905	35.9	10.0
1906	39.5	11.3
1907	39.9	11.6
1908	41.8	11.0
1909	39.4	11.5
1910	37.1	9.8

In the city of New York antitoxin came into general use early in 1895, when its free distribution to the poor by the Department of Health began. Largely by its use the total number of deaths from diphtheria and croup in every 100,000 of population in the Boroughs of Manhattan and the Bronx has been reduced since 1894 from 158 to 37, and bids fair to be still further lowered to 30 during the present year, while the case mortality has decreased from 29.7 per cent to 9.8 per cent, or one third its former amount. The table on the preceding page contains the official figures.

As with other serums, the beneficial action of the antitoxin of diphtheria is greater the earlier in the course of the disease it can be employed. This is very clearly shown by the following records furnished by the Brook Hospital of England for the eleven years from 1897 to 1907 inclusive:

PERIOD OF DISEASE WHEN ANTITOXIN WAS ADMINISTERED	PERCENTAGE OF DEATHS
1st day	0
2d day	4.29
3d day	11.24
4th day	16.89
5th day and subsequently	18.58

Besides its use as a curative agent, diphtheria antitoxin is employed very widely as a preventive. For example, if one child in a family is attacked with the disease, not only that child, but the other members of the family should at once be given antitoxin. If this be done, the spread of the disease will be checked and the total mortality will be diminished. The immunity conferred by a single injection usually lasts at least two weeks, and by subsequent administration it may be extended for a longer period.

The antitoxin of tetanus or lockjaw is prepared in essentially the same way as the antitoxin of diphtheria. Opinions have differed as to the degree of its value in those cases in which the disease has actually appeared, although it cannot be denied that it possesses some curative power, especially when injected into a vein. But there is no doubt of its great efficacy as a preventive. Its administration is an essential part of the treatment, in medical and surgical dispensaries, of injuries which are incidental to our customarily vigorous mode of celebrating the fourth of July, and many a patriotic American youth owes his life to antitetanus serum.

During the past century there has occurred in the United States and to some extent in foreign countries occasional outbreaks of a dangerous infectious disease, known popularly as spotted fever. It has destroyed many children, and left others pitiable physical and mental wrecks. From its epidemic character and the fact that its primary symptom seems to be an inflammation of the membranes or meninges covering the brain and spinal cord, it is called in medical circles epidemic cerebro-spinal meningitis. It is now known to be due to a specific bacterium, to which the name meningococcus is given. This organism is present in abundance in the nasal cavities of those ill with the disease. Its portal of entry into the body is the nose, and through the nose also it leaves the body, to infect, it may be, other unfortunate persons. A severe epidemic of this disease has spread over this country and a considerable part of Europe during the past six years, and various investigators have been stimulated to search for and to produce a specific serum for it. The most successful effort has been that of Flexner of the Rockefeller Institute in the city of New York. His serum is prepared by the injection into horses of both living and dead meningococci and an extract of them, which cause a reactive production of antibodies. These appear to be both antitoxin and opsonin, the latter being especially developed. The serum exerts also a destructive action directly on the living bacteria. When employed therapeutically it is injected into the spinal canal, and thus directly reaches the seat of the disease. It has been used for nearly four years, and it is estimated that it has reduced the mortality of the disease approximately from 75 to 25 per cent. Its success has been so pronounced that its preparation and distribution have now been entrusted to the New York Board of Health, and it takes its place beside the antitoxic sera of diphtheria and tetanus as an accepted therapeutic agent.

Flexner in this country and other investigators in other countries have now attacked another grievous infectious disease of young children, namely, infantile paralysis. It has been epidemic in this country for the past four years. It was probably brought here from the Scandinavian countries in 1907. The foci of the epidemic seem to have been New York and Boston, and from thence it has spread across the United States. Its mortality is not high, rarely exceeding ten per cent, but its baneful consequence is a partial paralysis of the arms and legs, resulting from a destruction of certain of the nerve-cells in the spinal cord. This paralysis is usually more or less permanent, and thus severely handicaps the individual in life's struggle. Here, as with other infectious diseases, comparatively little advance had been made until the illuminating method of animal experimentation began to be employed. Two years ago it was shown that the disease could be transmitted to monkeys by inoculating them with an emulsion made from the infected spinal cord of a child who had died of the malady, and that thereby typical cases of it could be produced. Thus the investigation began. The disease can now be readily transmitted by inoculation from monkey to monkey. Its virus appears to contain a living organism, and not simply a toxin. Its germ has not been identified, but from the fact that it can pass through the fine pores of the finest porcelain filter, it is inferred that it is one of the most minute organisms. The virus is exceptionally resistant and potent: even $\frac{1}{1000}$ of a single cubic centimeter of it, when injected after filtration into the brain of a monkey, suffices to produce paralysis. The disease is highly contagious, and, as in epidemic meningitis, the germ enters and leaves the body through the nose. It can be carried from place to place by house flies. One attack often confers a long-continued, if not a permanent immunity. This appears to be due to the presence of antibodies in the blood. By the employment of a suitable serum the onset of the paralysis can be delayed and often wholly prevented in a certain proportion of infected monkeys. Such a discovery hopefully points the way to the possibility of obtaining an effective serum for use with human beings, and active efforts are now being made toward this end.

A certain degree of success has attended the use of serums with erysipelas, puerperal fever, scarlet fever, typhoid fever, dysentery, and the plague, but none of these have yet come into extensive use. Various attempts have been made to produce serums for pneumonia, tuberculosis, and many other infectious diseases. But while some investigators report favorable results, these are not yet such as to warrant the general use of this method.

In certain other pathological conditions success has attended the use of specific serums. Here the principle of treatment is the same as with the germ diseases, for the pathological agent is a toxic substance which is capable of inducing the formation of antibodies. Thus, while arsenic, strychnine, and morphine do not stimulate such production, on the other hand certain vegetable poisons, such as abrin, ricin, and crotin, do so. Moreover, a serum has been produced which seems to diminish the virulence of hay fever. Considerable attention has been given to the preparation of serums against the venom of poisonous snakes, which in India alone are responsible for the death of 25,000 persons annually. A considerable degree of success seems to follow the use of antivenene, prepared by the French pathologist, Calmette. This appears to protect against the evil effects of the bite of the cobra. India possesses a variety of poisonous snakes, and a serum that is effective against the venom of one is probably not efficient against another: each serum seems to be strictly specific for its own poison. If this is so, it would appear necessary for the bitten victim to catch his snake and carefully determine its species before knowing which serum he ought to use. The difficulties in the way of this procedure are obvious. The hope has been expressed, however, that it will yet be possible to obtain a universal serum for snake bites.

While the serum method of treating infectious diseases has thus already accomplished much in a few important diseases, and will, without doubt, accomplish much more, its failures in other diseases have turned many investigators to seek the desired goal by means of vaccines. The principle involved in vaccination consists in introducing into the body of the patient not antibodies, as with serums, but rather specific substances which are capable of stimulating the body cells to activity in the production of antibodies. These specific substances may be, as in smallpox and rabies, a weakened or attenuated form of the same species of micro-organism, or, more usually, they consist of virulent germs, which, however, have been killed before the injection. Once within the body

H

they disintegrate, and the chemical substances thus released act upon the body cells, causing the cells to produce and cast out into the blood antibodies. In many cases, at least, these antibodies are opsonins. The living germs absorb them and become the palatable prey of the leucocytes. It is not altogether clear why the dead organisms thus artificially introduced are more efficacious than the living ones already present, but such seems to be the case.

Investigators have been encouraged to turn to vaccination by the great success that has attended the specific treatment of smallpox. Smallpox is a very ancient disease, and until recent years it has played a conspicuous rôle in history. For many centuries it was one of the great unconquered enemies of the human race. It was almost as inevitable as birth and death. It spared neither high nor low. Wherever numbers of people traveled they carried the disease with them : the crusaders spread it over Europe ; Spanish seamen brought it to America. In some manner, now unknown, in the centuries before the beginning of the Christian era, inoculation began to be practised in the Orient. This consisted in introducing under the skin of a healthy person some of the contents of a pustule from a person having smallpox, and thus deliberately inducing the disease. Thus begun, it usually ran a mild course, and conferred upon the patient a permanent immunity. In the early part of the eighteenth century the wife of the British ambassador to the Turkish Empire, Lady Mary Wortley Montagu, during her stay in Constantinople, became interested in inoculation, and not only submitted her children to it, but caused its introduction into England. Thence it spread to America. Inoculation was a courageous procedure, and, though effective, it was crude. It occasionally was the means of conveying other diseases ;

with each case it provided a new center of infection; the course of the disease in an individual was at times severe; and occasionally it terminated in death. A historic case was that of the eminent New England divine, Jonathan Edwards, who submitted to inoculation and died within one month after his inauguration as president of Princeton College. At the time when our American colonies were struggling for their independence, Edward Jenner, an English physician, was endeavoring to devise a more satisfactory method of combating this grievous disease. He is said to have learned from a milkmaid that those persons who contracted the mild cowpox were proof against the more severe smallpox. He investigated for many years, and in 1796 performed his first vaccination, using material from a human case of cowpox which had been contracted in milking. His success excited much interest, and his method soon came into widespread use. The causative agent of smallpox has not yet been identified beyond doubt, but it seems probable that it is a protozoan rather than a bacterium. It is believed that cowpox and smallpox are two different forms of the same disease, the germ in the former being weakened by its bovine life.

Wherever vaccination has been practised thoroughly, there is a nearly complete elimination of the disease. Thus in Sweden in the twenty-eight years previous to vaccination, smallpox killed 2050 persons annually out of every 1,000,000 of population; and in each of the forty years following only 158 persons. Germany inaugurated in 1874, and still retains, a model law, requiring all persons to be vaccinated in infancy and again in the twelfth year; and in 1899, out of a total population of 54,000,000 in the German Empire, there occurred only 28 deaths from smallpox. Its presence at all in Germany is due chiefly to its introduction by foreigners. Of the European countries Russia is still, in respect to this disease, a menace to the rest of the world.

Ever since vaccination began to be performed, there has existed among a small number of individuals, opposition to it. This is to be ascribed rather to perverseness than to reason. In the early days antivaccinationists claimed that the tendency of vaccination was to cause "bovine characteristics to appear in children; that they developed horns, hoofs, and tails, and bellowed like cattle." In recent years this class of people have denied the efficacy of vaccination in preventing smallpox — a denial that is overwhelmingly refuted by facts — and they assert that a variety of diseases result from the practice. In the early years, with the frequent habit of employing the virus taken from a human being and the none too cleanly treatment of the wound, there existed a certain element of danger of this kind. But this danger is now practically eliminated with the use of proper virus taken from young healthy calves, and of aseptic methods. In these days it is little less than criminal not to give to our children the protection which scientific medicine here offers.

The next step in vaccination for human diseases was taken by Pasteur with hydrophobia or rabies. While the victims of rabies have never been numerous, there has always existed a popular horror of it because of its frightful symptoms and the certainty of its fatal ending. I well remember my own and my playmates' youthful fear of the mad dog—the mad dog that was always possible but never met with. Many remedies have been recommended for its bite. Galen advised a preparation of the eyes of crayfishes, and Pliny, the elder, one of the livers of mad dogs. Not unfrequently those affected by the disease have been shot, poisoned, or suffocated. From classical times cauterization of the wounds has been the most frequent form of treatment. But no method was ever certain. Pasteur shared the popular feeling in regard to the disease, and in 1880 undertook its study. He never succeeded in seeing its germ, nor is it certain that any one has seen it, but he found that its seat is the brain and spinal cord. By the successful inoculation of the virus into rabbits he could increase its virulence up to a fixed point, and by removing from an infected animal the spinal cord and drying it, the virulence of the virus contained within it could be greatly diminished. This gave him the key to the practical application of his knowledge. If during the long incubation of the disease when introduced by means of the bite of a rabid animal, which averages some six weeks, he could effect within the body the growth of an attenuated virus, he might forestall the dreaded attack. He succeeded in doing this in dogs, and was able to afford them absolute and certain protection. Then came the extension of his method to a human being. Pasteur's hesitancy and agony of mind in this step have been told to the world. On March 28, 1885, he wrote to a friend: "I have not yet dared to treat human beings after bites from rabid dogs; but the time is not far off, and I am much inclined to begin by myself — inoculating myself with rabies and then arresting the consequences; for I am beginning to feel very sure of my results." On July 6 a young Alsatian lad was brought by his mother to Pasteur's laboratory, shockingly bitten by a dog, and though "divided between his hopes and his scruples, painful in their acuteness," he at last resolved to attempt to save the lad from what he felt would be a certain and terrible death. The first inoculation of a very weak virus was made, and day by day a preparation of constantly greater virulence was used. During the period of ten days' treatment "Pasteur was going through a succession of hopes, fears, and anguish." In the midst of it all he wrote to his son-in-law: "I think great things are coming to pass. . . . Perhaps one of the great medical facts of the century is going to take place." The boy left the laboratory well and apparently protected, but not until weeks after did peace of mind come to the man who had dared to bring to courageous completion his long research. In the autumn of the same year the story of his success had so far spread that he found himself beset on every side by requests for treatment which he could not refuse, and the extensive employment of his method was begun. Now it has become world-wide.

The procedure followed by the New York Board of Health in treating persons bitten by rabid animals is as follows in mild cases. In more severe cases stronger virus is used at first, and the treatment is continued for a longer time:

DAY OF TREATMENT	DURATION OF DRYING OF INFECTED SPINAL CORD IN DAYS	QUANTITY OF VIRUS INJECTED [1]
1	14 and 13 [2]	6 c.c.
2	12 and 11 [2]	6 c.c.
3	10 and 9 [2]	6 c.c.
4	8 and 7	6 c.c.
5	6	2 c.c.
6	5	2 c.c.
7	4	2 c.c.
8	3	2 c.c.
9	5	2 c.c.
10	4	2 c.c.
11	3	2 c.c.
12	5	2 c.c.
13	4	2 c.c.
14	3	2 c.c.
15	5	2 c.c.
16	4	2 c.c.

[1] Piece of cord ½ inch long, ground in 3 c.c. of salt solution.
[2] Cords dried for nine days or more may be substituted for these cords.

The most reliable statistics place the mortality of persons bitten by rabid animals in Paris before the introduction of Pasteur's treatment at 16 per cent, and the mortality of all cases treated at the Pasteur Institute at 0.6 per cent.

During the past decade various investigators, but particularly Sir Almroth Wright, have perfected a method of vaccination that has proved of great value in the prevention of typhoid fever. This consists of two, or sometimes three, inoculations, at intervals of several days, of a preparation of dead typhoid bacilli. An immunity extending over a period of perhaps three years is thereby produced. The treatment does not cure where the disease has already developed. It is preventive rather than curative, but even where it fails to prevent, it diminishes the severity and the mortality of the disease. It has been extensively employed in the British army in South Africa and India, and was introduced into our own army two years ago. British statistics show a decline in the number of cases from 5.75 per cent in the uninoculated to 2.25 per cent in the inoculated, and a diminution in case mortality from 26 per cent to 12 per cent. The results within our own army are even more striking. Among the troops, approximating 17,000 in number, who recently spent four months in Texas and southern California, the entire command having been inoculated, there were but two cases of typhoid, one of which occurred before the process of vaccination was completed. Among uninoculated civilians living in the same localities the disease was common.

Several vaccines against cholera have been prepared. That of Haffkine has been used extensively in India with pronounced benefit. The likelihood of becoming subsequently infected with the disease is thereby much diminished, and though, in those attacked subsequent to the protective inoculation, the percentage of fatality is nearly as great as in the uninoculated, there is no doubt whatever about the protective value of the treatment.

Haffkine's vaccine against the plague, which also has been used with large numbers of persons in India, is even more successful. The Indian sanitary commissioner says of it in his report for 1904: "That its value is great is certain; not only does it largely diminish the danger of plague being contracted, but, if it fails to prevent the attack, the probability of a fatal event is reduced by one half." Haffkine's figures for nearly 200,000 cases show a diminution of case mortality from 60 per cent to 24 per cent.

Vaccines have been tried as curative rather than preventive agents, with promising results in pneumonia, chronic cases of dysentery and diphtheria, and in various localized affections, such as abscesses. Beginning with Koch's tuberculin in 1890, a considerable number of vaccines have been devised during the past twenty years for the specific treatment of tuberculosis. They all have raised hopes and have had their advocates. Many of them have proved to be of little or no value. It is now recognized, however, that certain tuberculins are really curative, especially when they are employed in the early stages of the disease or in cases which are not advancing. They have also been used successfully in detecting its presence.[1]

Hiss has recently attacked the infectious diseases boldly by a new method. Recognizing that the white blood cells seem to possess within their bodies substances that are capable of neutralizing the bacterial poisons, he reasoned that if these substances could be supplied in quantity to an infected body, this larger stock of its own weapons would enable it to cope

[1] For a fuller discussion, see p. 126.

more successfully with the hostile germs. He has put his theory into practice. From the injection of aleuronat into the chest cavities of rabbits an abundant accumulation of leucocytes results within a few hours. These are withdrawn, water is added to them, and the extract of their substance is ready for injection into infected organisms. Many experiments on animals have warranted the extension of the method to man, and, while it is still in the experimental stage, beneficial results have been observed in pneumonia, erysipelas, epidemic meningitis, and various affections caused by staphylococci.

The discoveries which scientific medicine has made in recent years in the realm of the infectious diseases are now bringing to solution the long debated and puzzling problem of immunity. Certain diseases which are common in animals never, or very rarely, appear in man; in other words, man possesses an immunity to them. This is true of rinderpest, a disease prevalent in some countries among cattle, of dog distemper, and of chicken cholera. Particular individuals, too, appear to be immune to certain human diseases that may attack other individuals. This is strikingly illustrated by the differences among races in respect to certain diseases. The negro race is largely immune to yellow fever. Recovery from an attack of an infectious disease has long been known to bring with it a certain degree of immunity from a second attack. Thus a person who has suffered from smallpox is rarely attacked again by the disease. The protection which typhoid fever, yellow fever, scarlet fever, and measles offer is usually a life protection, although in the case of measles and typhoid fever this is not so assured as with smallpox. We now know that by the aid of serums and vaccines it is possible artificially to produce an immunity. With serums this immunity is of brief duration, lasting, for example, after the administration of diphtheria antitoxin only from two weeks to one month. How long it lasts after the use of vaccines is largely unknown. Its duration, however, is probably always less than that of the immunity acquired by an attack of the disease, and it varies with individuals. Thus it is popularly believed that vaccination against small-pox protects the individual for about seven years, but the protection may last for twice that period, or may be at an end within a single year. The protection offered by vaccination against typhoid fever, cholera, and the plague has been variously claimed to last for from six to eighteen months, or in the case of typhoid for at least three years.

In the light of what we have learned concerning bacteria, we can interpret many of these facts. Immunity appears to be due to various conditions. The body cells may not possess a chemical affinity for the toxins given off by the micro-organisms — in the language of Ehrlich, they may not possess proper receptors — and hence the toxins may never be able to enter into the cell substance and poison it. On the other hand, while possessing proper receptors, the body cells may possess at the same time the power of producing sufficient antibodies to ward off an attack of the disease. Such an immunity may be antitoxic, bacteriolytic, or phagocytic, according as the defensive weapons are antitoxins, antibacterial substances, or opsonins. As I pointed out in the preceding lecture, the body naturally makes use of these three methods in different degrees with different diseases. Scientific medicine, in its efforts to aid the body, while endeavoring to follow nature's lead, has succeeded in doing so in only a partial degree. Thus, while nature's method of combating diphtheria and tetanus seems to be through both antitoxins and opsonins, man has so far achieved striking success with those diseases only by the aid of antitoxins. With cholera and the plague, antibacterial substances appear to constitute nature's chief medium, while at present opsonins are man's. With typhoid fever man's success has been obtained in the same way as that of nature, through the agency of opsonins and leucocytes.

But scientific medicine has learned a method of preventing infectious diseases that is often more efficacious than the treatment of the infected individual. This consists in keeping the germs away from the individual. This is in fact the chief office of the public hygiene and sanitation, of which we hear so much in these modern days. The sources of drinking water may frequently be controlled, and contamination may thus be prevented. The simple storage of water in reservoirs is a means of purification, and is probably the most common method employed by cities in providing their inhabitants with a pure water supply. Water may be filtered on a large scale, and thus contaminating germs may be removed. This plan is now followed by the cities of London, Berlin, Hamburg, Lawrence in Massachusetts, and Albany in this state. For the home, efficient house filters, such as the Berkefeld and the Pasteur, are now readily obtained, and the boiling of water is efficacious. The problem of pure milk for the multitude is not easily solved. While milk is reasonably pure within the udder of the healthy cow, it always becomes contaminated in the process of removal, and, being a liquid mixture of easily digested food-stuffs, it is an excellent medium for the multiplication of bacteria. Even the certified milk obtainable in the city of New York contains on an average from 1000 to 5000 bacteria in every cubic centimeter, and the same quantity of ordinary milk obtainable in the shops frequently holds during hot weather several millions. More than two hundred varieties of bacteria have been found in such milk. While many of these are probably innocuous, experiments show that the feeding of milk heavily laden with bacteria to young children endangers their health, and even their lives. The one practicable method of destroying bacteria present in milk is that known as pasteurization, which, when properly performed, consists in heating the milk to a temperature of approximately 60° C. (140° F.) for some twenty to thirty minutes. This is sufficient to destroy the germs of tuberculosis, typhoid fever and diphtheria, and many other organisms, and does not materially affect taste, nutritive properties, and digestibility. Pasteurization is practicable for the educated consumer, and it may prove to be so on a large scale by a municipality. But it alone does not suffice, and the rigid inspection of dairies also appears to be essential to the securing of suitable milk for the multitude. The spread of rabies may be most efficiently prevented by the muzzling of all dogs for a definite period and the examination of all alien dogs introduced into the country. This is most readily practised in a restricted area. By this method England has practically eliminated rabies from her territory, and hence needs no Pasteur Institutes. Plague may be in part prevented by the destruction of rats. The most practicable means of eliminating malaria and yellow fever consists in destroying the possible breeding-places of mosquitoes. The same is true, but to a less extent, of typhoid fever and cholera in relation to the common house fly ; and the present crusade against this pest is worthy of all encouragement.

The proper attitude of society toward bacteria-carriers is not easy to determine. At present no form of treatment seems to insure the complete destruction of the bacteria with which they are afflicted.   It would be difficult to convince law-makers that such persons ought to be placed in detention, and yet there seems no reason to doubt that they constitute a source of menace to public health.   But society can and ought to see to it that every case of a developed germ disease, however mild it may be in the individual, is largely isolated from human contact.   This should be done even with such apparently trifling ailments as "colds," which, there is reason to believe, may harbor the germs of more harmful conditions.   Every case of an infectious disease may be a center for the infection of others, and, by its isolation, the possible evils arising from it may be obviated.   By such intelligent coöperation society can aid scientific medicine in the ultimate banishment of one of the chief causes of human misery.

VI

THOSE who have had sufficient persistence to follow the lectures of this course so far must necessarily have been impressed with the fact that a very large number and variety of medical problems, which have puzzled the world for centuries, have either been solved completely in recent years, or the way of their solution has been pointed out. With others medical science has not yet been so successful, and it is some of these others that I wish now to consider. I may say at once that present does not mean future absence of success. On the contrary, it means the opposite. I know nothing that is so conducive to a cheerful optimism in these present days as the pursuit of science. The laboratory is the habitation of buoyancy, enthusiasm, and hope. Its occupant has no moral right to be despondent, and, if he is so, there is surely something pathological in the activities of his brain-cells. Actually, however, one rarely meets with a pessimistic man of science. The experience gained in past advance but makes easier and more certain the way of advance in the future. Just as a bacterium within the body is a chemotactic center toward which leucocytes flock, so an unsolved problem in science draws investigators toward it. This is as true in medical science as elsewhere, and if a disease still progresses, it is a pretty sure sign that ere long something effective will be put in its way.

One of these unsolved problems about which we are now

hopeful is the great problem of cancer. To laymen the word is one of the most sinister in all medicine, bringing up a picture of a helpless being, harboring unwillingly a rapacious object, which eats its way through tissues and saps vitality until death brings the inevitable end. The picture is needlessly exaggerated, and yet it cannot be denied that it is sometimes true. Cancer is one of the strangest and apparently most lawless of vital phenomena. Picture to yourself the growth of the human body. From a single ovum there arises by continued division a mass of seemingly similar cells. Within this mass differentiation occurs, and the cells take on diverse appearances and groupings : some become muscle, some nerve, some gland, some bone, and some epithelium. Simultaneously the rudiments of organs appear, and functions begin to be specialized. The division of cells continues ; all proceeds in an orderly way ; each tissue finds its place ; and each organ, as it becomes perfected, becomes limited in size and diversity, so that it may work most advantageously for the good of the organism. At the age of about twenty years the body has largely ceased to acquire new tissue ; the period of active cell growth and division has nearly come to an end ; the existing cells have learned what they are to do ; and the real business of one's physical life proceeds according to law and system. But when one half of the normal space of life is passed, or even earlier than this, a strange thing may occur. At some point cell growth and division may start anew. But this time the process is not orderly, as in childhood, nor are the cells differentiated into tissues. It is unbridled, rapid, often tumultuous, and it rudely interrupts the orderly processes of life. The cancer-cells which appear are not like other cells, but have peculiarities of their own. The growing mass pushes its unwelcome way into the tissues, forcing them aside and pressing them back upon one another. In the center of the mass softening and degeneration may occur. Occasionally the cancer-cells may even act like cannibalistic phagocytes, devouring the cells of the organism that holds them. They make their way along the lymph-vessels and the blood-vessels, either by growth or after release from the main mass, and find new abiding-places, where they may become centers for additional growth. They seem to produce deleterious substances, which pass out beyond the scene of frenzied activity and poison the tissue-cells elsewhere. And thus the delicately coördinated body is made the scene of anarchy and riot. Anemia, weakness, and emaciation follow, and the final result too often is death.

What is the cause of this strange outbreak? In these days of disease-germs our first thought is that one of these low organisms has invaded the body, has found a soil favorable for growth, and is but exercising its innate right to prosper. Many attempts have been made to find the hypothetical germ for cancer. Many microscopes have been turned toward the new growth, and it has been searched through and through. Alien living objects have been met with in abundance. Now this organism, now that, bacteria, yeasts, protozoa, and other living things, and objects of unknown nature, have been found both within and without the cancer-cells and have been heralded as the long-sought germinal agent. But as surely as each discovery has been announced, so surely has it been discredited, and there never has existed any agreement as to the identity of the assumed agent. In view of many facts, it has now come to be believed by most pathologists that there is no such thing as a germ of cancer, and that the cause must be sought in a wholly different direction. So, too, cancer is not now regarded as an infectious disease.

Is cancer contagious? There has been in the past a wide-spread public impression that this dread disease may be transmitted from its victim to others by contact of the person or personal articles. Even physicians have believed this, and some have tried to support it by clinical evidence. The belief has even been so strong in some individuals as to stifle their innate sense of mercy, and to cause them to treat their afflicted fellow-creatures as outcasts to be shunned, and to make personal safety their ruling motive. Much has been written regarding the existence of cancer-infected houses, in which successive tenants have acquired the disease, and of its coexistence among persons living together. A careful examination of the evidence in the light of modern knowledge has now brought general conviction to the minds of those best qualified to know that the transmission of cancer by contagion does not occur. Statistics show that the occurrence of two cases within one family or one house is not more frequent than is demanded by the law of chance. The presence of a case within a family, therefore, need cause no fear of the acquisition of the disease by other members of the household. Much anxiety is often expressed over the possibility of the inheritance of the disease. Here again scientific medicine is reassuring. Cancer is not inherited, and statistics do not seem to indicate that there even occurs an inheritance of a predisposition toward it.

Cancer is comparatively rare among savage races. It is a disease of civilization, and as the storm and stress of civilized life become more turbulent, it seems to become more frequent. Apparently reliable statistics show that during the past half century it has increased in frequency over the more highly civilized part of the globe — in England, Scotland, Ireland, Wales, France, Germany, Holland, Norway, Sweden, Den-

I

mark, Switzerland, Italy, Austria, Australia, and the United States. The number of deaths from cancer in every 100,000 of population from 1890 to 1900 increased in England from 67 to 82, and in that portion of the United States in which there was adequate registration from 53 to 65. It occurs more frequently among women than men, a fact that is associated with the existence of the two most susceptible organs, the uterus and the breast. In organs common to the sexes it is more frequent among men. It is much more common after the age of thirty-five than before.

Cancers constitute one group of a large number of pathological growths, called tumors. If a tumor grows slowly, is sharply localized, consists of cells resembling normal cells, is not destructive to the surrounding tissues, and is comparatively harmless, it is called benign. A common example of such a growth is a wart in the skin. If, on the other hand, the tumor grows rapidly, spreads through and destroys the normal tissues, recurs when removed, and impairs the general health, it is called malignant, or a cancer. There exist several varieties of malignant tumors, and the term cancer is technically limited to that variety which is called carcinoma, and originates in epithelium. We shall here extend the term, as is often done, to include all malignant tumors. The cells of which a cancer is composed differ both structurally and functionally from normal specialized tissue-cells and appear to be more primitive, more embryonic in character.

A vast number of hypotheses have been proposed regarding the place, the manner, and the causative conditions under which cancers arise. It has been suggested that they have their origin in minute islands of primitive cells, actual remnants of the embryo, which were left unchanged when the differentiation of tissues occurred, lie dormant during all the years of childhood, youth, and early adult life, and later burst into unbridled activity. This was the view of the great German pathologist, Cohnheim. It has been suggested that the forerunners of cancers are groups of cells that have become misplaced or separated from their proper physiological continuity with other cells. It has been suggested that the first step in the growth of cancers is a degeneration of normal cells into cancer-cells; there is probably truth in this notion. It has been suggested that the cells destined to give origin to the cancer are sports, the offspring of cellular mutations. It has been said that the cancer-cells are those that have hitherto lived a normal life, but have now lost their habit of work and gained a habit of growth. Perhaps the sudden growth is only a manifestation of normal forces that have hitherto been held in restraint, and are now released; or these forces may have suddenly become increased beyond their normal bounds. All these and many other ideas regarding the nature of cancerous growth have been proposed and are now being actively discussed. External cancer appears to develop frequently in localities in which there has been long-continued inflammation or irritation. Thus an unhealed and constantly irritated wound, such as in the lip of an inveterate pipe-smoker, may become the seat of a cancerous growth. Sailors occasionally develop cancer as the result of the continued action of light on the skin. Long exposure to Roentgen rays is sometimes followed by the disease. It is widely believed, likewise, that internal cancers result from previous irritation; that, for example, an ulcer in the wall of the stomach is often a forerunner of a more serious cancerous growth.

It is hoped that much light will be thrown upon the genesis of cancer by a method of study that has been introduced within the past year by Carrel and Burrows and their associates at the Rockefeller Institute for Medical Research and is now being employed in various laboratories. It consists in growing the cancerous tissue in glass outside the animal body. A drop of the plasma of fresh blood is placed within a small shallow glass chamber, and is allowed to coagulate. A small piece of a cancer removed from the body of a man or a lower animal is placed within this nutrient liquid. The preparation is covered with glass, sealed tightly, and laid in an oven, which is kept at a uniform temperature equal to that of the living body. Under the influence of the warmth and abundant food, the remarkable power of growth possessed by the cancer-cells asserts itself. Soon they appear on the edge of the tissue. Many of them migrate outward. They multiply rapidly and push themselves out in long radiating lines into the clear plasma, and the extension of the cancerous mass is revealed even to the naked eye. Within twenty-four hours the area of the new growth has far surpassed that of the original fragment. The latter may even be removed, and the growth still continues. With the microscope each step in the process may be followed with ease.

While a cancer upon the surface of the body may be seen in its early stages, one of the difficulties attendant upon its presence within the interior is that of detecting it before it has become grossly obvious. Facts have recently been discovered which indicate that the cancer reveals its presence by the appearance in the blood of certain characteristic substances. While the existence of these substances does not seem to be confined solely to cancerous conditions, there is reason to think that in them we have a valuable auxiliary, although not an infallible aid, in the diagnosis of this disease.

Let us suppose that a cancer has appeared in an individual, and has been duly discovered. What is to be done? The most common procedure is to call in the surgeon and have him cut out the offending object; and of all known methods of treatment this is the most generally efficacious. If it be done in the early stages of the growth, before the tumor has become complex and has spread far from its place of origin, and if care be taken to remove it completely, without leaving remnants to act as centers of future infection, the surgical operation may be wholly effective and forever avert future trouble. But a late resort to the surgeon's knife, or a slovenly operator, although the main mass of the tumor may be removed, may only hasten the fatal ending. It may often happen, however, that it is not practicable to resort to surgery. Sometimes the disease has progressed too far, has permeated too much of the body tissue, or has seriously involved essential organs; sometimes it has so attacked the surface of the body that surgical removal would result in excessive disfigurement; sometimes the patient possesses ineradicable objections to surgical treament; and sometimes the physician has reasons for believing that a better way than through surgery can be employed. Hence methods have been devised with a view of destroying the new growth *in situ*. These methods are rendered practicable by the fact that the cancer-cells appear to be more sensitive to destructive agents than are the normal cells, and hence may be killed while the body cells among which they lie remain uninjured. Various destructive agents have been employed — caustic chemical substances, such as caustic potash or arsenious acid; the excessive heat of the surgeon's cautery; excessive cold, such as may be obtained from liquid air or frozen carbonic acid; the electric current; X-rays; and radium. All of these agents have been used abundantly; all have their enthusiastic advocates; and probably all are of some degree of value, although opinions differ greatly both as to their comparative merits and the circumstances under which they should be employed. There is, however, a general consensus of opinion among leading men of medicine that treatment by drugs accomplishes no more than a relief of specific symptoms, and is never curative.

During the last decade the investigation of cancer has taken on a wholly new aspect, because of the fact that it has been found possible to transplant certain varieties of malignant tumor from one animal to another. A bit of tumor is taken from the body of an animal in which it may have appeared spontaneously, is transferred to another animal, and there is engrafted within the tissues, where it adheres and proceeds to grow. Thus is made possible the method that is most effective in studying the phenomena of nature, the method of experimentation, in which the phenomenon can be produced at will and its conditions can be controlled. It is interesting to observe the reaction on scientific investigators of the discovery of this fact with regard to tumors. Eagerly and enthusiastically and hopefully they have turned toward the new field that has thus been opened up. Money has been contributed; new laboratories have been founded; old laboratories have been reorganized; other researches have been laid aside; and a concentrated, forceful move to solve the cancer problem has been inaugurated. Of institutes or laboratories for the investigation of cancer special mention should be made of those in Copenhagen, Frankfurt, Heidelberg, Berlin, Paris, London, Buffalo, the Rockefeller Institute for Medical Research in this city, and the Universities of Columbia, Cornell, Harvard, and Pennsylvania. The latest foundation, and one of the most liberal, is the George Crocker Fund, recently bequeathed to Columbia University.

Those who began the new line of investigation are Leo Loeb of this country, and Jensen of Denmark, who in 1901 independently demonstrated the possibility of employing animals effectively for such work.

Ten years of this experimental work have not solved the problem of cancer, but have contributed knowledge that is full of importance and promise. One result already evident is that the conditions of the growth of cancers are probably very delicately balanced. Thus only a few varieties of tumor may be transplanted at all, and these to only a few individuals of a few species of animals. Mice and rats are most susceptible to their growth, and have been employed for most of the experimental work. An illustration of the delicacy of the balance under which they grow is found in the fact that a certain variety of tumor which is very virulent for the mice of Berlin will not grow in the mice of Christiania. Moreover, if the susceptible variety of Berlin mice be bred in Christiania, they soon lose their susceptibility and become resistant to the same tumor. It is possible that this is due in part to a difference in the food supplied to the animals in the two cities: mice in the laboratory in Berlin are fed chiefly on fat and protein, those in Christiania on carbohydrate. Such a fact naturally suggests the probability that cancer will not grow in the bodies of human beings unless the nutritive conditions for such growth are exactly right. What these nutritive conditions are remains still to be discovered, but it is being shown that the growth of tumors under glass can be accelerated and diminished by various chemical and physical alterations of the medium in which they live.

The most promising of all the discoveries that the experimental method has yielded is the fact that a resistance or immunity to a tumor may be artificially produced. Occasionally an animal will recover spontaneously from a spontaneous or engrafted tumor. The cause of such recovery is unknown. This has its counterpart in the human body, where cancers occasionally recede and disappear of their own accord. When it occurs in an animal, or even when a tumor is merely present, it frequently follows that a second tumor cannot be made to grow in the animal's body: by the influence of the first growth the body has acquired an immunity to further foreign growths, not only of the same variety, but even at times of other varieties as well. The immunity thus acquired through a feeble tumor often protects against one of much greater virulence. Whether immunity to tumors, like immunity to bacterial diseases, is due to the production of antibodies by the body cells, or is to be explained otherwise, is not yet certain. If antibodies are formed, they would probably exist in the blood, and we might expect to find that the blood of such an animal possesses curative powers. With one variety of foreign growth, which is believed by many to be a tumor, this has actually been proved to occur: blood that has been taken from an animal that has recovered from such a growth and put into the vessels of another animal which possesses a similar growth has been found to make the latter to disappear. Such a fact may be explained on the hypothesis that in the growth of tumors protective antibodies are actually formed by the body cells. But certain facts, acquired also by animal experimentation, do not seem to agree with this interpretation, and indicate rather that acquired immunity to tumors may be due to a consumption of the food that is essential to their existence. Further work is needed along these promising lines of research; but whatever the explanation of the immunity, the fact that an immunity may be acquired at all is most prophetic of the future discovery of a method of checking the growth of and the curing of cancer in man.

As might have been expected, various investigators in recent years have turned toward serums and vaccines with the hope of finding in them the desired curative agent. The composition of these has naturally varied with the theories on which their authors have proceeded. Thus, it has been observed that if an individual suffering from a malignant tumor is attacked by erysipelas, the tumor frequently recedes and may actually disappear. This suggests that erysipelas is in some way antagonistic to the new growth. One investigator, acting on this suggestion, has actually treated tumors by the injection of toxins derived from the germs of erysipelas, and has appeared to have a certain degree of success with one of the less malignant types of new growth. Others, believing in the parasitic origin of cancers, have prepared serums from various supposed causative organisms. Still others have employed vaccines prepared in various ways. For example, the actual substance of cancer-cells, killed, pulverized and rubbed up in liquid, has been injected into patients suffering from cancerous growths. Some of these preparations have apparently been successful in the treatment of animals, and perhaps in isolated cases with human beings. But no serum or vaccine has yet been devised that has achieved striking curative success with human cancers. All are still wholly in the experimental stage.

I have given you only a small fraction of the knowledge that scientific medicine possesses regarding cancer, and I have enumerated but a few of the many discoveries in this field that have resulted from the introduction of the new methods. The problem of cancer becomes larger every day. It has come to be realized that it is a broad biological problem, and that it can be solved only by a fuller understanding of biological laws. There are two material objects to be studied, the cancer itself and the body in which it occurs. There constantly occur physiological interactions between these two, and the nature of these interactions must be discovered. The prevention or the cure of cancer is the goal that is of most general human interest; and although the way is not clear, there is every reason to believe that this goal will ultimately be reached. Let us hope that the attainment of this practical end will not be forced to wait upon an understanding of the many other features of this great problem.

While cancer is increasing in frequency, another of the major diseases of mankind, tuberculosis, is decreasing in most civilized communities. Thanks to the efforts of modern scientific medicine, the problem of tuberculosis is now well understood, and its solution is plainly in sight. Tuberculosis is an ancient malady. Even in the Hippocratic writings, five hundred years before Christ, there is a famous treatise on phthisis. There can be no question that the disease has been responsible for more human deaths than any other single agency connected with the life of man. Probably one human being in every seven dies of it. Its ravages are appalling in our own country, where a reliable and conservative estimate ascribes to it not less than 200,000 deaths annually. Moreover, it is estimated that we now have one million cases of it, and that its annual cost is from $150,000,000 to $200,000,000. Fifteen thousand persons die of it every year within the state of New York, and of these ten thousand die within our city. The results of autopsies indicate that practically all persons have at least a touch of it at some period in their lives. It may affect practically every organ of the body; it is masked under many guises and diverse names.

The lungs are the most common seat of the disease, and here the widespread name "consumption" is its most common designation.

The modern scientific epoch in the history of tuberculosis may be said to begin with the proof by Villemin, in 1865, of its infectious nature. It was not, however, until 1882 that the brilliant work of Koch demonstrated conclusively the bacillus that is the germ of the disease. There have existed much confusion and some difference of opinion regarding the relation of this bacillus as it occurs in man and domestic cattle respectively. It may now be regarded as conclusively proved that there exist two distinct types of the bacillus, the human and the bovine types, both of which are capable of causing tuberculosis in man. The genetic relationship of the two varieties is not known. The human type belongs primarily to the human body, and is the most common germ of the disease in adults. The bovine type belongs primarily to domestic cattle, and yet frequently thrives in the human body, especially in children. The relative proportions of the two in the human body are shown in the accompanying table. It is there seen that while the human type greatly predominates in man, the bovine type is common in children. Pulmonary tuberculosis, which is comparatively rare in young children, is probably almost exclusively of human origin.

RELATIVE PROPORTION OF HUMAN AND BOVINE TYPES OF THE BACILLUS OF TUBERCULOSIS IN 1038 CASES (PARK)

	HUMAN	BOVINE
Adults, 16 years and over . . .	65.0 per cent	0.8 per cent
Children, 5 to 16 years	9.5 per cent	3.0 per cent
Children under 5 years	15.5 per cent	5.6 per cent

The bacillus has the reputation of being a sturdy creature, very tenacious of life, but it is doubtful whether this reputation is wholly deserved. In the dried state it may remain quiet but living for several months. It will resist a dry heat of 100° C. (212° F.) for from twenty minutes to one hour, and a moist heat, as in milk or water, of 60° C. (140° F.) for perhaps fifteen minutes. Chemical germicides do not appear to kill it quite as readily as other pathogenic bacteria. It has a profound aversion to sunlight, the direct light of the sun sometimes killing it within a few minutes; when dried it may remain alive in darkened rooms for as long as ten months or more. Its favorable habitat, the human body, can by comparatively simple measures be made most distasteful to it.

Tuberculous human beings and tuberculous cows are the chief sources of infection for man. Tuberculous human beings give off sputum containing bacilli, which may be conveyed to other human beings, both adults and children, by coughing or by hands or lips, or may become dried and then transmitted through the air. Tuberculous cows produce infected milk, and this conveys the germs to children. Once within the body, the bacilli seek the most favorable localities, absorb food, and multiply. As they increase they do not swarm freely through the body, but prefer to remain localized in colonies in the lungs, joints, bones, membranes, glands, and other organs. They produce toxins, which are in some degree sent broadcast, but exert their deleterious action chiefly within the colonies. They stimulate the body cells to grow and produce unusual types of cells; leucocytes are attracted to the spot; and the strange admixture of native and foreign elements, supported by a fibrillar network and largely devoid of blood-vessels, constitutes the tubercle. Within it the body cells and the bacilli do not live amicably. Each force tries to destroy the other, and the invaders frequently have the greater success, causing the death and degeneration of the body cells. Then one of two things may occur. The tubercle may cease to advance, may develop an enveloping capsule, and may become hard, quiescent, and innocuous. On the other hand it may continue to progress; a constantly widening area of the surrounding tissue may become involved; other micro-organisms may invade the spot and lead to the accumulation of pus; if in the lungs, the growing tubercle may break through the wall of an air passage, and the débris of the degenerated tissues may be discharged, leaving a cavity; cavities of neighboring tubercles may fuse together; blood vessels may rupture and hemorrhage may result; and in the course of time the destruction of tissue and the interference with bodily functions may be so great as to cause death.

The body, however, possesses a very considerable power of resisting the attacks of the tubercle bacilli. A healthy, vigorous, well-nourished person, living in sunshine, breathing pure air, and exposed only occasionally to the germs, offers a poor soil for their growth, while, on the other hand, little air and light, underfeeding, fatigue, the constant use of alcoholic liquors, and frequent exposure to the bacilli are favorable to them. Yet, even after they have obtained a foothold, their course of development is very frequently checked before it has gone far. This probably happens in the great majority of individuals. The nature of this spontaneous cure is not yet understood. The body cells seem to be stimulated by the bacilli or their toxins to produce antibodies, but comparatively little has yet been discovered concerning such substances. Yet this lack of knowledge has not prevented investigators from searching in all directions for means with which to put a stop to this great scourge. The long list of drugs has been diligently searched, and it is now realized that they cannot act specifically on the bacilli themselves or their products. Such few drugs as are of use are of value in relieving the specific symptoms, such as the high fever and the cough, or in making the body more resistant in general to untoward conditions. As might have been expected, many serums and vaccines have been devised for the specific treatment of the disease. Of the serums those of Maragliano and Marmorek are the most prominent, but there is no general agreement that they or other serums are of real value. The vaccines are more numerous. While differing in certain respects, they are alike in consisting of some or all of the products of the bacillus. The whole world was startled in 1890 when Koch announced the results of his experiments with one of these vaccines, tuberculin, and it was widely believed that at last the long-sought cure for consumption had been found. But the world's expectations were greater than those of Koch. Too much was demanded of tuberculin. It was used by the competent and the incompetent, grossly, irrationally, and in cases that were beyond all aid. When the world learned, what Koch had always known, that tuberculin was not a universal cure for consumption, the world, even much of the medical world, turned upon and unjustly denounced both the remedy and its maker. But here again the pendulum swung too far. It was sure to go back, however, and so it has. Tuberculin — which word has now become the generic name for the more prominent tubercular vaccines — is prepared in various forms, which vary in composition and physiological action. It is being very widely used as a means both of diagnosing and of treating the disease. As a diagnostic agent its injection is followed by a rise of temperature if tuberculosis be present, and by no such reaction, or only a very slight one, if tuberculosis be absent. This test for the presence of the disease is now employed constantly with domestic cattle and frequently with human beings. As to the therapeutic value of tuberculin, those who have used it most intelligently testify to its worth. Thus it has been used with a considerable number of patients at the Adirondack Cottage Sanitorium under the skilful direction of Trudeau since 1890, with the result that, while in the incipient stage of the disease it seems to have made little change, of the moderately advanced cases those who have been discharged from the institution apparently cured number six per cent when untreated, and twenty-seven per cent when treated with tuberculin. Notwithstanding the partial success of tuberculin, it must be granted that the ideal specific remedy for tuberculosis has not yet been found, although medicine has by no means given up the search.

But fortunately for the human race tuberculosis, when compared with other infectious diseases, is peculiarly responsive to more general therapeutic measures. These constitute the now well-known hygienic-dietetic method of treatment. The three most pronounced features of this method are rest, both physical and mental, combined with carefully regulated exercise, liberal feeding, and an abundance of fresh air. A change of climate is sometimes valuable, but not essential. Life in a sanitorium insures a stricter adherence to the principles of this treatment than life in the home. Permanent improvement under it is never speedy; it may demand from three months to three years, and a cure may require still more time. Naturally the incipient or moderately advanced cases are more favorable than those that are far advanced. For wage-earners life in a sanitorium is often impossible. This fact should cause no despair, for the treatment of the disease in the home has abundantly justified itself, and here the dispensary and the visiting nurse have proved a blessing.

One of the most remarkable and most hopeful philanthropic movements that has ever been undertaken is the present campaign against tuberculosis, which has been stimulated directly by the achievements of scientific medicine. Many countries are engaged in it, but it has been most highly organized in the United States and the state and city of New York. For national work the National Association for the Study and Prevention of Tuberculosis is preëminent; for the state of New York the State Charities Aid Association; and for the city of New York the Committee on the Prevention of Tuberculosis of the Charity Organization Society. There now exist in the United States nearly 500 associations, 300 special dispensaries, and 400 special sanitoria and hospitals, with nearly 25,000 beds, all devoted to specific antituberculosis work. During 1909 the various state legislatures appropriated a total of about $4,000,000 for the campaign. Each year shows an increase over all preceding figures. Although this work must ultimately have a preventive effect on the disease, it has been inaugurated for too short a time to afford undoubted statistical results — unless the following figures are so interpreted.

NUMBER OF DEATHS FROM TUBERCULOSIS PER 100,000 OF POPULATION IN THE STATE OF NEW YORK

YEAR	URBAN DEATHS	RURAL DEATHS
1907	189.4	126.6
1908	184.4	124.3
1909	175.5	121.1
1910	165.5	121.3

The table shows that the decrease in the mortality of this disease during the past four years has been more rapid in urban than in rural communities. The cause of this is not clear, unless it be ascribed to the greater efficiency of the antituberculosis measures employed in cities.

While the forces engaged in this work aim to provide treatment for those unfortunate persons who are afflicted with the disease, it is recognized that the surest way of solving the problem of tuberculosis is to prevent its extension, and energy is now expended chiefly in this direction. It is realized that the most prolific centers of infection are the home and the crowded places of business, where the infected person comes into intimate association with the uninfected and the bacilli may readily be transferred from the one to the other. It has been estimated that fifty-one per cent of all children in tuberculous families acquire the germs of the disease. The control of the germ is, therefore, the essential factor in the prevention of the disease. I have mentioned the fact that the total mortality from tuberculosis is gradually diminishing. This is strikingly shown in some of those communities in which the segregation of advanced cases in institutions has been practised, as, for example, in England, Scotland, and Wales, and it seems reasonable to associate this manner of dealing with the disease and the decrease in its death-rate as cause and effect. The present efforts of those who are directing the war against it are being expended partly in educating the people concerning it, and partly in securing the establishment of hospitals for advanced and incurable cases and of sanitoria and dispensaries for those who may still be cured. When public opinion will sanction the segregation of all dangerous cases, and when hygienic conditions of living have become such as to prevent susceptibility to the disease,

K

the days of this ubiquitous and deadly bacillus will be numbered.

Pneumonia is an acute infectious disease which still offers a serious problem to scientific medicine. The pneumococcus seems to be the chief causative agent in both the so-called lobar and lobular types of the disease, but several other microorganisms may be present. The fact that the pneumococcus is one of the most universal and ordinarily innocuous inhabitants of the air passages of healthy persons indicates that its presence alone is not the sole essential factor in the incidence of the disease. The body must contribute favorable conditions for the bacterial growth. In lobar pneumonia the bacteria pass into the blood, but are localized chiefly in the lungs, where they cause severe inflammation, resulting in the clogging of the alveoli or air-cells with foreign substance, and serious interference with the respiratory exchange between air and blood. Intensely poisonous bacterial toxins, which appear to be endotoxins rather than exotoxins and incapable of stimulating the body cells to the production of antitoxins, are given off, probably on the death of the germs, and seriously affect the heart and other organs. Opsonins are probably produced, and the lungs become the ground of a fierce contest between leucocytes and germs, in which the individual too often succumbs. Antibacterial serums have been prepared, but have not met with great success. Vaccines, especially those prepared from a culture of the germs taken from the patient himself, appear to act favorably in certain cases. But no specific treatment is markedly effective, and the pneumococcus continues to take its abundant toll of human lives.

Cancer, tuberculosis, and pneumonia illustrate well the variety and complexity of the conditions that scientific medicine has to meet in its campaign against disease. Questions of physiology and pathology, of bacteriology and pharmacology, of chemistry and physics and general biology, of psychology, ethics, and sociology, have to be asked and answered. The unsolved problems are still many, and all encouragement should be given to the devoted men who are laboring to accomplish their solution and the manifold blessings that will thereby be conferred upon mankind.

VII

THE most dramatic chapter in medicine is that of surgery. An old English proverb runs, "A good surgeon must have an eagle's eye, a lion's heart, a lady's hand." If this were true in the days of medievalism, it is much more so now. The transfer from the medieval to the modern in surgery has taken place within the memory of living men. It is true that even before this generation boiling oil was no longer poured into wounds to assist the healing process, but there were two features that still were prominent, as they had been prominent from neolithic times. These were the pain of the operation and the uncertainty of its outcome, owing to the almost inevitable septic conditions that followed it. These two features have now been almost wholly eliminated by the discovery of anæsthesia and asepsis, the two most important general surgical advances of our time.

That the early surgery was a matter of agony for the patient can easily be conceived and is abundantly attested by literature. We read of "the excruciating tortures and writhings and shrieks of patients on the operating table." An eminent American surgeon has written of operations before anæsthesia: "Prior to that time a surgical operation was attended with horrors which those who live in these days cannot appreciate. He was the best surgeon who could perform any operation in the least possible time. The whole object of

132

new methods of operating was to shorten the period of frightful agony which every patient had to endure. Every second of suffering saved was an incalculable boon. To submit to any operation required then a heroism and an endurance which are almost incomprehensible to us now. All of the more modern, deliberate, careful, painstaking operations, involving minute dissection, amid nerves and blood-vessels, when life or death depends on the accuracy of almost every touch of the knife, were absolutely impossible. It was beyond human endurance quietly to submit one's self for an hour, for an hour and a half, for two hours, or even longer, to such physical agony." Even those who operated felt the horror of it. It is related of the famous English surgeon, Cheselden, that "he always before an operation felt sick at the thought of the pain he was about to inflict." Various attempts were made to allay the pain. The ancient Europeans used mandrake, the Chinese and East Indians hasheesh. Later other drugs were employed, among them liberal doses of opium or of alcoholic drinks. But all these were far from ideal. The situation, however, was completely and quickly changed by the success of an operation in the year 1846, at the Massachusetts General Hospital in Boston, when the eminent surgeon, Warren, painlessly removed a tumor from the neck of a man who had been put under the influence of ether by the dentist, Morton. This operation created great excitement in the surgical world, and, among other results, stimulated Sir James Simpson of Edinburgh to experiment with a stronger anæsthetic, chloroform. His success caused the introduction of chloroform into surgical procedure in the year following that of ether. The use of these agents soon spread far and wide, but their universal employment did not occur without the inevitable opposition to innovations.

Such opposition came from two sources. Certain men of medicine objected to the new practice on the singular grounds that "pain during operations is, in the majority of cases, even desirable, and its prevention or annihilation is for the most part hazardous to the patient;" "pain should be considered as a healthy indication . . . an essential concomitant with surgical operations . . . the natural incentive to reparative action." But more singular objections than these were raised on religious grounds. It was argued that to avert pain was to thwart the will of God, and biblical passages were brought forward to support the contention. To controvert the various objections, even the defenders of anæsthesia were forced to singular lines of argument. Thus, Sir James Simpson wrote as follows: "Those that urge, on a kind of religious ground, that an artificial or anæsthetic state of unconsciousness should not be induced merely to save frail humanity from the miseries and tortures of bodily pain, forget that we have the greatest of all examples set before us for following out this very principle of practice. I allude to that most singular description of the preliminaries and details of the first surgical operation ever performed on man, which is contained in Genesis ii, 21. 'And the Lord God caused a deep sleep to fall upon Adam; and he slept; and he took one of his ribs, and closed up the flesh instead thereof.' In this remarkable verse the whole process of a surgical operation is briefly detailed. But the passage is principally striking, as affording evidence of our Creator himself using means to save poor human nature from the unnecessary endurance of physical pain. 'It ought to be noted' (observes Calvin, in his commentary on this verse), 'that Adam was sunk into a profound sleep, in order that he might feel no pain.'" Whichever party had the best of the argument, common sense prevailed, and the new era of painless surgery was quickly inaugurated. One early result of this was a great increase in both the number and variety of operations. Ether and chloroform have continued as the favorite general surgical anæsthetics, though nitrous oxide and other substances are sometimes employed. Still others are used to great advantage for the purpose of producing insensitiveness at the immediate site of the operation, and thus obviating the profound effects of an anæsthetic that pervades the whole body. Among such local anæsthetics cocaine is the most important. Of late years an entirely new method has been advocated for rendering insensitive the lower parts of the body. This consists in injecting a suitable drug into the lower portion of the spinal canal, where it temporarily paralyzes the outgoing nerves and even the spinal cord itself, and prevents the passage of nervous impulses to the brain. Cocaine, tropococaine, novocaine, stovaine, and other drugs have been so employed. Notwithstanding the fact that the method has been subjected to much and varied criticism, it seems to have a definite field of usefulness.

But with the discovery of practicable anæsthetics the battle was only half won. The operation itself had lost much of its horror, but the tragedy of the subsequent days was unchanged. There were the almost inevitable suppuration of the wound, the putrefaction and sloughing off of tissue, the sickening odor, the high fever, the danger of hemorrhage, the slow healing, the complications of blood poisoning, erysipelas, gangrene, and tetanus, the physical and mental anguish, and the uncertainty of the final outcome. The mortality from major operations was from fifty to one hundred per cent. The opening of the abdomen, the chest, or the skull was undertaken only in extreme cases, and "was almost equivalent to signing the death warrant of a patient." The wounds of two bloody wars, our Civil War and that of France and Germany, testified to the impotence of septic surgery. But Pasteur's studies had already proved that fermentation and putrefaction were due, not to "gases, fluids, electricity, magnetism, ozone, things known or things occult," but solely to microscopic living germs. The English surgeon Joseph Lister, holding a professorship at Glasgow, had become acquainted with Pasteur's work and, a firm believer in what certain sceptics called "mythical fungi," reasoned that if the germs caused putrefaction elsewhere they could do the same in wounds. He therefore conceived the idea of bathing wounds with, and applying to them dressings of, carbolic acid for the purpose of killing whatever germs were already present. He applied this to several cases of compound fracture with marked success in inducing healing without suppuration, and thus in 1867 antiseptic surgery had its birth. To Lister, who continued for years actively to experiment, has been granted great honor in all civilized countries, and he has had the privilege of seeing surgery completely revolutionized by the stimulus of his labors. In the rise of bacteriology it has been shown that the suppurations, putrefactions, blood poisonings, erysipelas, and other untoward sequelæ of the early surgical operations were caused not by anything already present in the body of the patient, but by bacteria, which were introduced into the wound at the time of the operation. These came not so much from the air as from the surgeon and his implements. The warm, moist, nutritive surfaces afforded most favorable conditions for growth and multiplication. The bacteria throve, some of them spread throughout the body, and each species produced its characteristic symptoms. Thus the old-time surgeon, with his hands, his instruments, his sponges, his lint, and his bandages, was teeming with disease germs, and the wonder of it all is that the mortality resulting from his unclean, even though well-intentioned, work was not greater than it proved to be.   Not until Pasteur and Lister pointed it out did civilized man know what constitutes real cleanliness.   Lister later introduced the method of maintaining throughout the surgical operation a delicate spray of carbolic acid in the air over the wound.   Still later the use of germicidal agents during the process of operating was found to be unnecessary.   Strict cleanliness was proved to be sufficient, and antiseptic surgery gave place to the aseptic surgery of to-day.

The absolute sterility, or freedom from bacteria, of all things that come into contact with the wound is the *sine qua non* of the successful surgical operation of the present day. In order to insure this, the patient, the surgeons, the attending nurses, the room, the operating-table, the instruments, the ligatures, and the dressings are elaborately prepared. Mechanical cleansing, chemical germicides, and heat are employed in removing or killing the bacteria.   All sheets, towels, cotton wool, gauze, and bandages that may come into contact with the tissues at the site of the operation, as well as the clothing of the surgeons, assistants, and nurses, are sterilized by being submitted to a high degree of heat in a specially prepared oven.   All instruments are thoroughly boiled in an antiseptic solution, and are then dried on sterile towels or are laid in a sterile liquid.   Sea sponges, which were formerly used freely, have now given place to sponges of sterilized gauze; lint and old linen have been replaced by sterilized cotton wool and muslin; sterilized catgut has become the most common material for ligatures.   The patient's skin at the site of the proposed operation is thoroughly and repeatedly scrubbed with cleansing antiseptic agents. The surgeon removes his outer clothing, and dons a sterilized gown which covers his body. His head is encased in a sterilized cap and frequently a sterilized mask, which covers the face except the eyes, and prevents any contamination from the mouth and nose. The hands and forearms are submitted to most thorough and prolonged washing, are subsequently soaked in antiseptic solutions, and are then covered with sterilized rubber gloves. Surgical assistants and nurses undergo a preparation scarcely less elaborate than do the surgeons. When the environment is thus freed from bacteria, the operation proceeds, practically without the aid of further germicides.

With pain and bacteria eliminated, the way was open for surgery to develop along rational lines, and the advance of the past forty years has been unexampled. No portion of the body is longer regarded as inaccessible to the surgeon's instruments. The most striking improvements have involved the three great cavities of the body — the abdomen, with its many organs of nutrition, the chest, with the lungs and heart, and the cavity of the skull, containing the brain.

The abdomen can be freely opened without the former inevitable peritonitis resulting, and can be thoroughly explored. The stomach can be opened; foreign bodies that have been swallowed can be removed from it; wounds in its walls can be repaired; ulcers, cancers, and other tumors can be removed; when the incoming and the outgoing openings, those of the œsophagus and the intestine respectively, have become constricted, they can be enlarged; if the œsophagus has become permanently closed, a new entrance into the stomach can be made from the outside through the abdominal wall, and food can thus be introduced; if the stomach has become too greatly dilated, tucks can be taken in its wall; if it sags, its ligaments can be shortened, or it can be stitched to the wall of the abdomen; parts of it can be removed; new connections can be made between it and the intestine — a procedure that is now followed in a considerable variety of conditions; and lastly, in a number of extreme cases, the stomach has been removed *in toto*, and the œsophagus and the intestine have been joined directly. Operations analogous to those of the stomach can be successfully performed on the intestine, wounds being sewed up, portions of it several feet in length being removed, new connections being made between adjacent parts; and, if necessary, external openings can be made from it through the body wall. The intestinal operation that has excited the greatest amount of popular interest is undoubtedly that of the removal of the vermiform appendix, which has raised this humble little organ to a position of surgical prominence that is altogether out of proportion to its physiological importance. The appendix is a small tube, branching out from the large intestine near its beginning and closed at the farther end. In certain of the lower animals, as in the rabbit, it is large and is stored with partially digested food. In man it is some three and one half inches in length and one quarter of an inch in diameter, and is a degenerate organ, of no great importance functionally. It is a pity that it has not long since met the fate of other of nature's remnants. It is peculiarly prone to infection, and it is probable that bacteria are the chief factor in the onset of inflammation which we call appendicitis. The most common bacterium is the colon bacillus, the universal bacterium of the large intestine, although septic organisms, pneumococci, and tuberculosis bacilli are frequently found there. The accusation that is commonly heard against seeds

and other foreign bodies as the cause of appendicitis seems
to be unjust.   While a mild inflammation of the appendix
may at times be allayed by external treatment, it is now
agreed by most physicians and surgeons that removal is the
one effective remedy, and that it should not be long delayed.
The operation has been performed for about twenty-five years,
and is done with great ease and rapidity, a skilful operator
requiring only from fifteen to thirty minutes in uncompli-
cated cases.   It is not regarded as dangerous if performed
early in the course of the disease and by a competent
surgeon.   Under such conditions its mortality does not
appear to be above two per cent.

The liver has the most abundant supply of blood-vessels
of any single organ of the body, and it contains one quarter
of all the body's blood.   Hence it might be supposed that its
surgery would be difficult because of hemorrhage.   Here,
however, nature's provision that the pressure of the blood
within the hepatic vessels is comparatively low assists the
surgeon, with his artificial means of preventing a loss of blood.
A variety of operations on the liver can be successfully performed, such as the repair of injuries, the draining of abscesses
and of cysts due to parasites, and the removal of tumors.
In these and other operations it is sometimes necessary to
remove parts of the organ itself, and considerable portions
of it have thus been successfully taken away.   Nature's
generosity to mankind is shown in the fact that the remaining
portion suffices to perform for the whole body all the important hepatic functions.   It happens occasionally that the
liver settles down below its proper place or becomes freely
movable.   In such conditions its suspensory ligaments can
be shortened ; it can be sewed to the abdominal wall ; or its
upper surface can be scarified and made to adhere to the

diaphragm; by these various devices the liver can be restored to and anchored in its proper place.

One of the body's organs that frequently causes trouble is the gall bladder. This is prone to become the site of the formation of gall stones, which are concretions composed largely of cholesterin, one of the waste products of bodily activity. They frequently follow an attack of typhoid fever, and the cholesterin is then deposited about the typhoid bacilli which have tarried within the gall bladder. The presence of gall stones excites inflammation within the bladder, and their involuntary expulsion through the hepatic duct is often accompanied by excruciating pain. Their surgical removal is desirable, and within the last decade the operation has become common. It consists either in opening the gall bladder and removing the stones alone, or in taking away the entire bladder itself. The mortality from this latter operation is less than two per cent, and the absence of untoward effects shows that the organ and its function as a storehouse for bile are not necessary to the body's needs.

The spleen may likewise be totally removed without detriment to health. Considerable portions of the pancreas may safely be taken away. The kidneys are subject to a considerable variety of disorders that demand surgical treatment. Such treatment includes sewing a kidney to the tissues of the back, the repair of wounds, cutting into it, draining it, the removal of calculi, and the removal of the kidney itself, either in whole or in part. The removal of both kidneys is fatal.

Surgical operations on the chest or thorax and its organs are rendered difficult, first, by the great liability of the parts to infection, a liability much greater than that of the abdominal organs, and secondly, by the peculiar mechanical conditions that are presented. The cavity of the chest is divided by delicate membranes into three separate compartments : the right and left pleural cavities, occupied by the right and left lungs; and between them the mediastinal space, containing the heart, the large blood-vessels joining it, the thoracic lymph duct, the œsophagus, the trachea, and certain large nerves. By the respiratory movements of the walls of the chest and the diaphragm below, the pleural cavities and the air passages of the lungs are alternately enlarged and diminished, and air is alternately drawn through the nose or the mouth and the trachea into the lungs and expelled by the same route. At all times during health, even in extreme expiration, the lungs are distended, now more, now less, yet they always entirely fill the pleural cavities. But when the chest wall is punctured, as by a wound, or a lung is ruptured, as by the breaking down of a tubercle, air rushes into the corresponding pleural cavity, and the lung collapses like a torn balloon and becomes partially incapable of performing its respiratory function. This condition, while dangerous, is not fatal if the opposite lung and pleural cavity are uninjured. In that event respiration, though diminished, still goes on, and if the injury can be healed, the thoracic air is absorbed and the affected organ later resumes its rôle. A surgical operation on a lung involves entrance through the thoracic wall, and the consequent hazardous interference with respiration. Various devices have been introduced to overcome this. Sometimes an intermittent or a continuous stream of air is forced under pressure into the trachea and the lungs, and thus respiration is maintained artificially during the operation. Sometimes the body of the patient and the surgeons are placed in a pneumatic cabinet, through an opening in one wall of which the patient's head protrudes. Thus he breathes air, as normally, under the prevailing atmospheric pressure. The air in the cabinet, however, is maintained at less than this pressure, and thus both pleural cavities can be safely opened without danger. While operations on other thoracic organs are now varied and numerous, operations on the lung substance itself are still comparatively limited. Nevertheless pathological growths within the lungs are beginning to be successfully removed, and in various other diseased or injured conditions portions of the pulmonary tissue have been taken away. Even the surgical treatment of tuberculous lungs is coming into favor. The present outlook for an extended pulmonary surgery is distinctly hopeful.

The living beating heart is commonly thought to be a most delicate organ, the slightest interference with which may lead to serious consequences. Physiologists, however, have long been accustomed to experiment elaborately upon the hearts of animals, and have learned that they are really very hardy. Even the hearts of warm-blooded animals will withstand much manipulation within the body, and may be removed *in toto* and retain their activity for many hours or even days. Notwithstanding this, it has not been easy to overcome the feeling that the human heart must be left untouched. For many centuries its wounds were regarded as necessarily fatal, and it is only within a period of about fifteen years that surgeons have come to realize that this vital organ is not outside their legitimate province. "The road to the heart," says a graphic writer, "is only two or three centimeters in length in a direct line, but it has taken surgery nearly twenty-four hundred years to travel it." It should be added that the route has finally been pointed out through animal experimentation. Exposure of the heart in man is a comparatively simple procedure, which does not interfere with its action and does not necessarily involve the opening of the pleural cavities. Once exposed, the heart can safely be handled, turned about for examination on all sides, and even be lifted out of its nest. Wounds of the heart can thus be definitely located, and are now sewed up, as are wounds in other and less vital organs. Unless bacterial infection occurs, or the loss of blood or the shock is too great, the proportion of ultimate recoveries is considerable. Foreign bodies, such as needles, knife-blades, and bullets, have been successfully removed from the heart. But all such operations are merely the beginning. Investigators are now experimenting on animals with some degree of success in the endeavor to devise methods by which more intricate pathological conditions, such as the abnormalities of cardiac valves, the heart's cavities, and blood-vessels can be corrected. These methods frequently require the temporary cessation of the flow of blood through the heart. One limitation to protracted operations arises from the fact that if the circulation of the blood be thus interrupted for more than four or five minutes, serious and permanent degenerative changes occur in the brain. Nevertheless, as knowledge increases, we may confidently look forward to a considerable extension of cardiac surgery.

One of the striking instances of the many protective adaptations with which the body is provided is afforded by the bony cranium covering the brain. The bones comprising the body of the skull are not only arched — the best mechanical device for resisting external pressure — but are extremely hard. The brain, which is essential to the maintenance of an orderly life, is unusually well guarded against injury from without. Nevertheless, it is not wholly free from disorganizing agencies. The most resistant of arches may yield and the hardest of bones may be fractured, and thus the brain within may be made to suffer from direct injury to its tissues, from the presence of foreign objects such as bullets, from hemorrhages, or from pressure of broken bones or escaped blood. So, too, infective bacteria may enter through external wounds or by the way of the blood or the lymph, and set up abscesses or inflammations. And lastly tumors of every variety may develop within the brain substance. In many of these cases operative relief is demanded, and here scientific surgery has achieved some of its most brilliant results. The opening of the skull cavity by trephining is the first step in the operation. Curiously enough trephining was practiced in prehistoric times, as is shown in ancient skulls. This must have been done with stone instruments, and probably for both injuries and brain diseases. At times it was doubtless associated with the theory that diseases are due to demons which departed through the hole in the skull. In the days of Hippocrates trephining was well known. One hesitates to think of the slight success of such a heroic operation when performed with primitive means. In these aseptic days it has been greatly perfected. It is a quick, simple, and reasonably safe procedure to cut through the scalp and with the circular trephine to saw from the skull a button of bone, thus exposing to view the membranes of the brain and beyond them the brain itself. If a larger field is required, a larger piece of the bone covering is removed, care being taken to preserve it for returning to its place at the end of the operation. Perhaps the most striking use to which this method is now put is in the removal of brain tumors. For the exact location of such foreign growths a knowledge of the physiology

L

of the brain is necessary. Since the pioneer work of the ingenious German physiologists, Fritsch and Hitzig, in 1871, it has come to be known that the body nerves are connected with localized groups of nerve-cells within the brain, each group constituting a center for a particular part of the body. Thus the eyes are represented in the brain by certain centers, the ears by others, the muscles of the fingers, of the arms, of the vocal organs, by still others, and so on throughout the organism. If the nerve-cells in one of the centers be destroyed, the activity of both the center and its corresponding bodily organ ceases. If the center or its outgoing nerves be unduly pressed upon, the tissues may either be stimulated to an activity that is greater than normal, or, on the other hand, may cease to act. In either case the activity of the bodily organ keeps pace. Thus, one of the causes of blindness may be destruction of, or pressure upon, the brain center of sight; and one of the causes of the paralysis of the arm may be destruction of, or pressure upon, the center that controls the arm's movements. On the other hand, pressure upon a sensory center may, through undue stimulation, cause unusual sensations, or upon a motor center an abnormally prolonged contraction or spasm of the muscles involved. Such destruction of or pressure upon the parts of the brain may be due to cerebral tumors, among the important symptoms of which are the affected bodily movements and sensations. By a careful observation and analysis of these, the surgeon may be guided to the source of the trouble in the brain, and may then remove the pathological growth, thus removing its manifestations. If the substance of the brain center has been actually destroyed by the tumor, or is so involved in it that the removal of the one necessitates removal of the other, other portions of the brain may often apparently take on the lost function, and the bodily organ may thus be restored to normal activity. Brain surgery has invaded the field of the long mysterious disease known as epilepsy, which is manifested by distressing bodily convulsions, or "fits." While the remote cause of the epileptic condition is complex and unknown, there is no doubt that the convulsive attacks result from excessive activity of that portion of the cerebral cortex which controls the body's movements. It is even possible to produce experimentally in animals a convulsion like that of epilepsy, by exposing the motor area of the brain and stimulating it by an electric current. In many cases of epilepsy there exists a lesion of this motor region due to injury or disease. An early surgical operation, which removes the irritating agent, has afforded benefit in a considerable number of cases.

The work of the surgeon is not confined to the correction of deformities, the repair of wounds, and the removal of tissue. He frequently finds it necessary to supply deficiencies. The earliest known instance of this is the transfusion of blood. In the early years it was a favorite dream that through the replacement of blood, one might cure diseases, invigorate the enfeebled, and overcome moral obliquity; and in the latter half of the seventeenth century blood transfusion from animals to men for healing purposes began to be practised in Europe. From that time for two hundred years it had its enthusiastic advocates, but its all too frequent failures prevented its becoming universal. The objection to the use of blood from an animal that is far removed from man in the zoölogical scale is owing to the fact that, on being introduced into the human vessels and mingled with human blood, the foreign, and to some extent the native, corpuscles are promptly destroyed, and thus the benefits of the operation are nullified. This destruction of alien corpuscles is but one instance of the defensive power of the body against foreign substances — a power which here might appear to be acting contrary to the body's own interests, and which would perhaps have been ordered differently by us, if we, instead of nature, had had the body's fashioning. However that may be, the human body seems to be intolerant of any but human blood. This fact has led to the frequent practice, in cases of need, of introducing into the veins a solution of common salt. This is often distinctly beneficial, especially when there has been great hemorrhage. But the ideal circulating liquid is healthy human blood, and within the last decade methods have been perfected by which its transfusion can be safely effected. A preliminary test with a few drops of blood should be made of the compatibility of the blood of the individual who is to become the donor with that of the recipient, in order to be sure that the mixture will not result in a destruction of corpuscles. The operation consists in exposing and opening an artery or a vein of the donor, frequently the radial artery of the forearm, and uniting it to a vein of the patient by the delicate stitching together of their coats, by an intervening glass or metal tube, or by some other method that avoids clotting. The blood, pumped by the donor's heart, is then allowed to flow slowly to the recipient until a suitable quantity has passed. The loss to a healthy vigorous person of a considerable quantity of blood entails no serious consequences, and it can be replaced within four or five days, while, except in a few cases, that which is transfused finds in the recipient's body a congenial home and proceeds to perform its customary duties. Some of you will recall the striking case of two years ago in this city, when the infant daughter of a physician was saved from death by the process of transfusion. The baby of four days suffered from the disease called hemophilia, which is characterized by a constant oozing of blood from the capillaries of the body. Every method of stopping the hemorrhage that was known to medicine was tried in vain, and the child at last reached a state of weakness that meant its death within a few hours. As a last resort the father resolved to try the effect of transfusion. An artery in his own arm was stitched to a delicate vein in his baby's leg, and for ten minutes his blood flowed into her body. The fresh, healthy, red fluid was retained, and proved to be of the right composition. The child revived, and now owes her vigorous life to the knowledge and the skill of the scientific surgeon. Transfusion is now practised in a variety of conditions, such as hemorrhage from various causes, shock, jaundice, as a preliminary to a surgical operation that promises to prove dangerous to the patient, and in poisoning by illuminating gas, in which the blood, thoroughly saturated with the carbon monoxide of the gas, is unable to take up oxygen.

A second instance of the transplantation of deficient material is that of skin grafting, which has now been performed very successfully for twenty-five years. Where, because of disease, surgical operations, or accidents, parts of the body have become denuded of their skin, it is possible to replace it. One of several methods consists in shaving thin ribbons of the superficial layers of healthy skin from a smooth area, such as the inside of the thigh, either of the individual himself, or of another donor. These ribbons consist of the epidermis and a portion of the dermis, and may be five or six inches in length and one and one half inches in width. They are carefully spread over the denuded surface, where they soon become firmly adherent; blood vessels penetrate their lower layers; the growth of cells begins; and within a few days a layer of fresh tissue has made its appearance. This gradually increases in thickness, and in time the new skin assimilates itself to the old. A patch of negro skin grafted upon a white person becomes white; white skin on a negro becomes black.

A new era in reconstructive surgery seems likely to be inaugurated through experimentation that is now being carried on in the transplantation of whole organs. This work is being performed on animals, but its growing success seems to point the way to its ultimate extension to human beings. A number of experimenters in various parts of the world are engaged in it, and notable results have been obtained in this city by Carrell, of the Rockefeller Institute for Medical Research. It has been found possible, for example, to remove from one animal a segment of an artery, even the aorta, the largest artery of the body, and replace it by a similar piece of artery taken from another animal. The transplantation is successful even when the piece has been kept in the cold for several weeks. A piece of artery from an animal of a different species has even been employed. Thus successful transplantations of arteries have occurred from the rabbit, the cat, and even from man to the dog, and from the dog to the cat. But, so far as I am aware, the experiment has not yet been tried of transplanting from a lower animal to man. Segments of veins have been used to replace segments of arteries. In this case an interesting transformation in structure takes place. The piece of vein in its new position is subjected to a hitherto unwonted pressure from the blood, but proves itself equal to the emergency. Instead of yielding, the connective tissue in the thin wall grows and causes a marked thickening and strengthening of the vessel, and thus the new piece adapts itself to its elevated arterial dignity. The future application of such facts to human surgery may possibly be made in a variety of defective arterial conditions. If, for example, the wall of an artery becomes weak in a particular spot, a bulging outward may occur, constituting an aneurism. This may greatly increase in size and ultimately burst, causing a fatal hemorrhage. The new experimental work indicates the possibility of removing such a section of artery and replacing it with a healthy piece which had previously been obtained from the body of a man killed by accident. It is not yet known whether the artery of a lower animal can be so employed.

Successful transplantations of thyroids, parathyroids, ovaries, spleens, and kidneys have been performed in animals. Carrell has transplanted from one cat to another, in a single mass, the two kidneys, their arteries and veins, with the adjoining parts of the aorta and the vena cava, the nerves and the nervous ganglia of the kidneys, the entire ureters, and the part of the wall of the urinary bladder through which the ureters enter. The organs attached themselves to their host's body, and performed their functions well, although death from unknown causes occurred after five weeks. The partial success of such a complex operation is most encouraging. Carrell has also succeeded in transplanting the entire leg below the knee from one fox terrier to another. One leg of one dog was carefully amputated, its blood was washed from its vessels by a suitable solution of inorganic salts, and the leg was laid aside. The corresponding leg of the second dog was then amputated. The first leg was then fixed to the stump of the second; bones were joined to bones; muscles to muscles; nerves to nerves; arteries to arteries; veins to veins; and skin to skin. The blood, which throughout the operation had been prevented from escaping, was then admitted to the newly acquired limb and was found to circulate. Normal healing was complete at the end of fifteen days. Most of this work of transplantation has been performed within the past five years. It is thus in its infancy, and it is impossible to predict what its outcome will be. It opens, however, a wide field of possibility and suggestiveness, and it is not improbable that it will point the way to unique developments in human surgery.

In the preceding lecture I have referred to the recent achievements in the growth of tumors outside the body.[1] By a similar method other tissues may be made to grow. Harrison, of Yale University, first demonstrated the growth of long nerve-fibers from nervous tissue taken from an embryo frog. The method has now been extended at the Rockefeller Institute under Carrell and Burrows to other tissues of young chicks and both young and adult dogs and cats. As with tumors, bits of normal tissue are placed on glass slides in the clotted plasma of blood, the preparations are then sealed and placed in a warm chamber, and, in the course of a few hours, active cell growth and division begin along the edges of the tissue and extend out into the plasma. The growth is less rapid than with tumors under similar conditions. Nerve-fibers, cartilage, connective tissue, bone, skin, cornea from the eye, mucous membrane, and some of the tissues of the spleen, thyroid, and suprarenal glands, pancreas, and kidney have thus been cultivated successfully. Endeavors are being made to discover the manifold conditions under which such growth occurs, and influences that will accelerate and retard it. It is not possible at present to foretell how far this kind of investigation will carry us. One practical result may be the discovery of means by which the healing of wounds, which is now left largely to nature, may be greatly acceler-

[1] See p. 115.

ated.   In the moods of our greatest optimism we may be
permitted to dream of far greater and far more wondrous
achievements.

Remarkable as has been the advance of surgery in recent
years, there is no reason to believe that the end is yet in
sight.   Surgery is no longer merely an art of skilful cutting
and sewing; it has risen to the higher level of a science.

VIII

THE RÔLE OF EXPERIMENT IN MEDICINE. THE PUBLIC AND THE MEDICAL PROFESSION

OUR review of some of the features of modern medicine has, I trust, made it evident that within the past century, and largely within half that period, medical science and art have advanced with a speed incomparably greater than at any previous time. There has indeed been a second veritable renaissance. Instead of proceeding in a circle, as in Bacon's time, the advance has been in all directions outward into the unknown from the great mass of that which was already known. The path of science is always devious. Science essays this way and that, and rarely reaches its goal over the course of a straight line. But the path of medical science was never straighter than it has been during this modern epoch. The cause of this unprecedented progress is as complex as is that of any other movement of civilized man; but the most powerful single factor is undoubtedly experiment. Ancient medicine is characterized preëminently by philosophical speculation and empiricism; modern medicine by experimentation. The ancient physician was content to observe phenomena as they existed under their natural conditions, to interpret them in accordance with a philosophical system, and to treat disease in the light of what his system and past experience had taught him. The modern physician does not rely on a philosophical system. Like his forerunner, however, he, too, observes phenomena under their natural conditions; but he goes further than this and alters the conditions, and thus he obtains an alteration of the phenomena and a new standpoint from which to view them. He may apply to the cure of disease past experience, it is true, but it is past experience that has been put to the test of modern experiment. Moreover, by the aid of further experiment he pushes out into the unknown, sees disease from unusual standpoints, and devises new and hitherto unsuspected methods of dealing with it. If he forms a working hypothesis, it, too, has to be submitted to experimentation, for men of medicine have little patience with a new idea that has no experimental evidence in its favor.

But what do we mean by experimentation? We obtain our knowledge of the phenomena of nature from observation by means of our special senses, which modern physiology tells us are more in number than the traditional five. Through the gateways of these six or seven senses we may look out and see what nature is doing. But the more we have learned by such simple observation, the more eager to learn we have become, and the more impatient of always waiting for nature to present her phenomena in her own chosen way. We have learned, moreover, that nature is not immutable, but that we can change the conditions under which she manifests herself. Thus, if nature shows us an object cold, we can make it warm; if it is dry, we can moisten it; if it contains certain chemical constituents, we can replace them by others; if it is a living object at rest, we can stimulate it to activity; if its processes are complex, we can resolve them into simpler ones. Thus we can voluntarily control nature's phenomena in a great variety of ways; we can control their beginning, their progress, and their ending; and in this way we can make them more accessible to observation. This is the essence of experimentation. It is the voluntary control or modification of natural phenomena. It is an artificial aid to simple observation. By means of it we can penetrate more rapidly and more deeply into nature's secrets than it would ever be possible for us to go unaided.

Some of the ancients performed experiments. Archimedes conceived the greatest of them all: "Give me where I may stand," he said, "and I will move the earth." It is doubtless well for us of a later generation that his condition was impossible of fulfilment. But Galen was less ambitious. He tied an artery of a living animal in two places, and on opening it between the ligatures found that it contained blood, and thus at once by a simple device he disproved the theory of all the centuries that had preceded him, that the arteries were air-tubes. Harvey, in Charles the Second's time, was fertile in experiments to demonstrate that the blood circulates. A century and a half later Haller cut the nerve connecting the spinal cord and a muscle, and demonstrated that the muscle is capable of contraction without receiving the hypothetical animal spirits from the brain. But experiment as the all-important method of acquiring knowledge did not permeate science until the nineteenth century, until men realized how inadequate for advance were both philosophical systems and unaided observation. One by one, various branches of medical science have come to realize that the experimental method is indispensable to their progress. Physiology was the first to appreciate this. Then followed pharmacology, pathology, and bacteriology; and lastly anatomy has come to see that a complete knowledge of structure can be obtained only through a knowledge, acquired experimentally, of the mechanism of growth. The achievements of the experimental method are already extraordinary, and its future possibilities seem almost inexhaustible.

Let me illustrate how this method is applied to-day to the study of a single organ, the heart of a higher animal. A knowledge of the structure of this organ should first be obtained by observation of the dead heart, dissecting it, and examining its tissues by the aid of the microscope. A comparative study of the hearts of a series of animals is valuable. It is desirable also to know how the heart has developed from its earliest embryonic appearance to its adult stage. It is obvious that without some preliminary knowledge of the way in which the heart acts, it is difficult to learn much of its physiology while it is still enclosed within the chest. One of the first experimental procedures is, therefore, to make it more accessible. Happily anæsthetics have simplified this. An animal, such as a dog, a cat, or a rabbit, is anæsthetized by means of one of the accepted general anæsthetics, ether or chloroform. The heart is not exposed at once, but the trachea in the neck is first opened and one end of a tube of glass or metal is inserted into the opening and fastened in place. Through this tube the vapor of the anæsthetic is readily administered throughout the subsequent course of the experiment, of which the animal knows nothing. The heart can then be exposed to view by cutting away the front wall of the chest and opening the pericardium. Because of the free opening of the chest cavity, the lungs collapse, and natural respiration becomes impossible. Through the tube in the trachea, however, a current of air can be pumped intermittently into the lungs, and this artificial respiration must be maintained thereafter. The heart can then be quietly and leisurely observed in activity. No one, however unimpressionable, can watch a living, beating heart lying before him, with its parts contracting and relaxing in perfect rhythm, alternately emptying and filling, hardening and softening, paling and blushing — no one, I think, can watch such an object without a profound feeling of admiration, on the one hand for its wonderful mechanism, and on the other for what scientific medicine has been able to accomplish in devising methods for its understanding. But direct observation of the heart *in situ* is only the beginning. Levers with writing points can be attached to its various parts, and their movements can be graphically recorded on moving paper in the form of waves, which reveal the force and the rate of the beats and any alterations in force and rate that may chance, or be made artificially, to occur. The heart can be connected with a delicate galvanometer, which indicates the electrical changes accompanying its beats. An artery can be opened and connected with a manometer, which measures and records the pressure within the artery and the pulse-beats, and gives a clue to the amount of work that the heart performs. The cavities of the heart can be connected with similar manometers, and their dynamic conditions can thus be revealed. The two kinds of nerves passing from the brain to the heart can be artificially stimulated and their actions can be observed and recorded — the one kind weakens, slows, and can temporarily stop the beats; the other strengthens and quickens them. The depressor nerve passing from the heart to the brain can be stimulated — it depresses the activity of the vasomotor center in the brain, and thus reflexly dilates the body's arteries and diminishes the arterial resistance against which the heart has to contend. The two kinds of nerves directly supplying the arteries can likewise be stimulated, the one constricting, the other dilating them, and thus the effects of varying blood-pressures can be recorded and studied. By stopping respiration temporarily the action of varying degrees of asphyxia can be stud-

ied. By comparing the chemical composition of the incoming with that of the outgoing blood, data can be obtained
concerning the effect of the heart's action on the blood, and
the metabolism of the heart muscle.   Metabolic products,
foods, drugs, poisons, and bacterial toxins can be injected into
the blood, and their varying actions on heart and arteries can
be observed.   The blood can be removed and replaced by
blood of a different composition, or by an artificial circulating
liquid, and thus the action of heat, cold, and various chemical
substances can be studied.   The action of the heart valves
can be interfered with, as happens in various diseases.   Other
diseased conditions can be produced and studied with an
exactness such as never can be hoped for in the intact body.
The heart can be wholly removed from the body, can be fed
with a nutritive liquid and be kept beating for hours under
artificial and easily controlled conditions, which make
possible the exact observation and record of many influences,
normal and pathological.   Parts of the heart can be removed
and studied in action, an experiment which simplifies the
investigation of certain problems, such as the nature of the
heart beats.   And so, in a thousand ways, undreamed of
by our predecessors and often incomprehensible to the
layman, we have acquired and are still acquiring knowledge
of the normal and pathological phenomena of this intricate
organ.   Yet this is but a small part of the tale that may be
told.   There is no organ in the body, physical or chemical,
to which the experimental method is not applicable, and
from which secrets may not be wrung by its intelligent use.

Obviously the experimental method requires laboratories
in which the work may be carried on, and within seventy-five
years, beginning with Purkinje's physiological laboratory,
which was established at Breslau in 1839, such institutions

have sprung up throughout the world in all of the medical sciences. No other field of scientific work is now more active. Of great importance also are the innumerable clinics and hospitals that have been established. The latter half of the nineteenth century was especially rich in the founding of such institutions and the improving of those already existing. Clinics and hospitals are necessary adjuncts to the laboratories, since they offer opportunities for the application to human beings of the results of laboratory research, and, furthermore, serve as laboratories for such experimental work as can legitimately be carried out on men.

Of the innumerable varieties of experimental work now undertaken, it is obvious that a certain proportion cannot be performed upon human beings. No one is morally justified in removing from the body of a fellow-being a vital part, or endangering his life or well-being in any way for the purpose of experiment. For such work animals lower than man are employed, and these include a considerable variety of species, ranging all the way from the microscopic protozoa to the higher mammalia. The use of anæsthetics, as in human surgery, has quite altered the aspect of such work, and allowed a great extension of it. Animals are now employed for many varieties of physiological investigation, for determining the physiological actions of drugs, foods, and other chemical substances, for standardizing drugs, for devising new surgical operations, for the preparation of serums, for diagnosing certain diseases, for studying disease, and in teaching the elements of medical science to students. Many diseases can be experimentally induced in animals, and thus their causes, treatment, and cure can be more rapidly and effectively investigated than under the limitations of investigation in man. This is strikingly true of the infectious diseases. From a study of the conditions in animals one can pass to the observation of normal and diseased states in man with a host of preliminary questions already answered, and with a clear appreciation of how to proceed and what to do in order to understand and alleviate human conditions. The use of animals for experimental purposes has, in fact, been one of the most important factors in the rapid and efficient advance of scientific medicine.

In view of the great extension of the commendable humane movement of the past half century it is perhaps not surprising that opposition to the use of animals for scientific purposes has appeared in certain quarters and is hotly maintained by a few individuals. This opposition sometimes wilfully denies the value of animal experimentation in scientific progress; it sometimes assumes the extreme and ethically indefensible attitude of denying the right of man to use animals at all as experimental objects; and it has as its practical aim the establishment of legal restrictions against the practice. These vary in degree from slight limitations to total prohibition. The antivivisection view is psychologically of great interest. It rests on a low intellectual and ethical level, and exhibits in an elemental simplicity the qualities and the power of emotion. Its abnormal sympathy for animals blinds its possessor to a normal sympathy for human beings. It assumes the present existence of cruelty in laboratories. As evidence of such cruelty it either recites for the thousandth time one of a half dozen classic instances of experimental procedures that date from an early period before the use of anæsthetics became general, or it misinterprets or misquotes instances of modern procedure. I have been at considerable trouble to make a detailed examination of its literature, searching for the origin and the justification

M

of its oft-repeated phrases and its specific charges of cruelty, and I have found the literature wholly unreliable. Its misleading character has indeed often been pointed out, and has now, I think, became generally recognized. It should never be resorted to as a source of correct information regarding the modern laboratory. Many antivivisectionists are frequently sincere, and undoubtedly undergo great mental anguish over the supposed unwarranted sufferings of animals. But they are fighting a monster that does not exist. Effective anæsthetics are as universal in operations upon experimental animals as in those upon man. At the conclusion of an operation, if the existence of the animal's life is no longer required, he is painlessly killed ; if it is required, he is humanely cared for. If a disease is produced within his body, there is every reason to believe that because of his low mental organization he suffers far less than would a human patient under similar conditions. Opposition to animal experimentation has succeeded in Great Britain in placing the leaders of scientific medicine under severely restrictive laws and a constant suspicion which is degrading both to them and to their fellowmen and hostile to healthful scientific progress. The force of this opposition is now happily diminishing among the more intellectual classes in England. In the United States the antivivisection movement has never secured any considerable following, and no legislature has yet yielded to its fanatical demands. Nor is this to be expected. Scientific research has already brilliantly justified its claim that only through freedom from petty restrictions can it advance. Biological and medical research has demonstrated that it is humanitarian in the highest degree, both in method and in achievement. Men of medicine have been practically a unit in resisting opposition to such research, and this resistance

should be stoutly maintained if our present rate of progress
in scientific medicine is to continue.   In the interest of this
progress and of a broad humanitarianism, not only men of
medicine, but the public outside of the medical circle, should
jealously guard the freedom of scientific experimentation.

The increasing breadth of investigation in the medical
sciences is coupled with a broadening of those who partake
in it, and has enabled them to realize that theirs is a part
of a comprehensive biology.   In discovering the laws of
health and disease they are not simply saving human beings from death, but are contributing to the larger field of
the science of life.   Much investigation in medical laboratories
hence seems at first sight far removed from medicine.   Ehrlich injected dye-stuffs into rabbits, and observed what
tissues were most deeply colored.   There might seem no
possible relation between this strange proceeding and the
cure of disease, yet it led him to appreciate clearly that
specific drugs possess precise affinities for specific cells.
Thence he was led through a long series of experiments to the
discovery of that compound of arsenic, a single dose of which
may seek out with unerring exactitude and destroy every
Treponema in a syphilitic body, and thus put an end to a
loathsome disease without injuring the tissues in which it
thrives.   By a similar course he seems to have found an
equally effective and safe poison for the germs of sleeping
sickness.

I know of no more striking instance of an apparently
purely scientific discovery yielding large practical benefits
than that of Galvani and his frogs.   Galvani was a
physician living in the old Italian city of Bologna, and a
professor in its ancient university.   The electrical machine
was already long known, and Franklin had performed his

experiments on atmospheric electricity. Galvani became interested in the apparently trivial phenomenon of the twitching of the muscles of frogs' legs. He performed many and diverse experiments to ascertain the source of the stimulation. He proved that, contrary to expectation, the electrical machine was not necessary, nor was atmospheric electricity. But when he allowed a circuit to be completed through the frog's muscles, a brass hook attached to its spinal cord, and an iron trellis of his house, he always obtained a vigorous contraction of the muscles. This simple and seemingly childish experiment has brought in its train momentous results. In the first place, it was the beginning of a knowledge of animal electricity, which we are using daily for the interpretation of physiological phenomena, and, in some degree, for the diagnosis of disease. But, far greater than this, the use of two metals in Galvani's experiments suggested to Volta that in their dissimilarity lay the source of the electricity. He thereupon proceeded to experiment with metals, and evolved the voltaic pile, the first apparatus to generate a continuous electric current and make a study of its powers possible. The galvanic battery soon became a reality; experiment succeeded experiment; and to-day we have the electric light and the thousand uses to which electricity is put, direct descendants of an observation made by a physician in order to understand why frogs' legs twitch. The city of Bologna is properly proud of its citizen's achievements, and has not only inscribed his house, but has erected in one of its public squares a statue of Galvani, holding in his hands a tablet bearing an image of his preparation of frogs' legs. Discoveries like his — and such instances are numerous — show us that we can ill afford to decry scientific experiments that do not have an immediately obvious, practical application.   Of two men of science we sometimes hear the practical man praised as the man who does things, while he who spends his time investigating theories is looked upon as a dreaming idealist, whose discoveries may be interesting enough, but are of little use.   This attitude of mind is even found within the medical profession itself, but its short-sightedness has been demonstrated so often that it is less common there now than formerly.   It is one of the cardinal features of the anti-vivisection idea.   The sooner we free ourselves from such a narrow conception of scientific endeavor, and the more we encourage the freedom of research, the sooner will scientific medicine arrive at its goal.   The success of the practical man is largely due to the fact that he applies the principles which the idealist has discovered.

In the first lecture of the present course I spoke of the popular distrust of both the medical profession and its efficiency in curing disease.   Such distrust has always existed.   The literature of all ages is full of gibes regarding things medical. A chilly Greek epigram runs thus: "Marcus, the doctor, called yesterday on the marble Zeus; though marble, and though Zeus, his funeral is to-day;" and a Latin proverb affirms that there is "more of danger from the physician than from the disease."   Montaigne, who suffered from a common ancient malady, which the medicine of his time found hard to cure, at last became very tolerant of his trouble and his pain, but not of his inefficient sixteenth-century physicians. In his essays he has a famous chapter in which he expresses himself freely concerning them.   "Mine ancestors," he says, "by some secret instinct and naturall inclination have ever loathed al maner of Physicke."   "My father lived three score and fourteen yeares;   my grandfather three score and nine; my great-grandfather very near four score, and never tasted or tooke any kind of Physicke." "The very sight of drugs bred a kinde of horror in my father. . . . I see no kinde of men so soone sicke, nor so late cured, as those who are under the jurisdiction of Physicke. . . . A Lacedemonian being asked, what had made him live so long in health, answered 'The ignorance of physicke!' . . . A physition boasted unto Nicocles, that his Arte was of exceeding great authority. It is true (quoth Nicocles) for it may kill so many people without feare of punishment by Law." Yet it was not against physicians that Montaigne bore malice. "As for me I honour Physitions, not according to the common receiv'd rule, for necessitie sake . . . but rather for the love I bear unto themselves; having seene some, and knowne diverse honest men amongst them, and worthy all love and esteeme. It is not them I blame, but their Arte." A hundred years later that master of delicious comedy, Molière, ridiculed well the degenerate medicine of his time. It is related that the king once asked him how he got along with his physician, and he replied: "Sire, we talk together; he prescribes remedies for me; I do not take them; and I get well." Sganarelle, who was made a doctor in spite of himself, soon found it a profitable undertaking: "I think I had better stick to physic all my life. I find it the best of trades; for, whether we are right or wrong, we are paid equally well. We are never responsible for the bad work, and we cut away as we please in the stuff we work on. A shoemaker in making shoes can't spoil a scrap of leather without having to pay for it, but we can spoil a man without paying one farthing for the damage done. The blunders are not ours, and the fault is always that of the dead man. In short, the best part of this profession is, that there exists among the dead an honesty, a discretion that nothing can surpass; and never as yet has one been known to complain of the doctor who had killed him." Now the art of the twentieth-century doctor is a very different affair from that of his forerunner of four hundred or three hundred years ago, yet Montaigne's and Molière's commentaries, as do those of the ancients, have a curiously modern sound ; so much so indeed that one cannot refrain from thinking that much of the present distrust of the medical profession had its rise in tradition. Traditional criticism can always find sympathetic ears. It long ago became the custom to deride the doctor. Montaigne and Molière inherited it, and so have the critics of to-day.

Next in order among the causes of the present distrust of medicine I would place ignorance. And here, first and most important of all, is the appalling ignorance which people possess of their own bodies and their bodily processes. If asked to locate his heart or his stomach, the average man would probably place the one in the middle of his left chest cavity, and the other in the middle of his abdomen. Of their functions he would be chary of expressing an opinion, but he knows that the heart is related in some way to the circulation of the blood, and that the stomach receives food and digests it, or at least attempts to digest it. He has less knowledge of the purpose for which his liver exists, except to make him "bilious" or to get "sluggish" or "torpid" or "out of order." He is usually not aware of the fact that he even possesses a pancreas, and when assured that such an organ really exists, he is quite at a loss to know of what possible use it can be to him. He has no clear idea of the arrangement of the nerves in his body, nor of the way in which they perform their tasks. He cannot analyze a reflex action. The solar plexus to him is only a place in which to hit his opponent. A supposedly intelligent lady, after listening to one of Huxley's lucid lectures on the brain, asked him if he would kindly enlighten her about one point which she had failed to grasp, namely: whether the cerebellum is inside or outside the skull? A vasomotor nerve would be a poser for the average man, as would the tricuspid valve, the thyroid gland, the pancreatic duct, lymph, trypsin, the pylorus, and the mode of seeing and hearing, though he might talk glibly of his "system," his "economy," his "constitution," and his "pores" — all of them echoes of a prehistoric physiology. Of how to maintain his health he thinks he knows much. He says that this food "agrees" and that food "disagrees" with him; and with much feeling, but little reason, he ascribes particular sensations to particular foods. He remembers the identical draft which caused his present "cold." He believes in exercise, but does not take it. But if he has so little clear conception of what goes on within himself normally, how does he behave when disease comes, for of pathology he knows less than of physiology? He feels certain symptoms, but he does not understand their diagnostic significance. He knows not whether they are important or unimportant, or whether or not they demand a doctor's knowledge. He trusts blindly to the hope that if he neglects them they will pass away. If they persist, he diagnoses his own disease and attempts to treat it. If at last he is forced to appeal to the doctor, he learns that of the real nature of his disease he knows practically nothing, except what the doctor may tell him. Largely because of ignorance, he shrinks from a surgical operation until the extreme condition has arrived. He will submit to the taking of innumerable drugs, but for what purpose they are prescribed, of the physiological action of the components of a prescription, he has no conception. And so, from the beginning to the end, there is ignorance, crass ignorance, of the body, and what the physician can do for it.

A third cause of distrust of medicine lies in the inability of the physician to do certain things. We all have had personal experience of this. In considering it we should bear in mind that the common soldier fighting in the ranks is never the peer of his commanding officer. The great body of the medical profession has not the scientific knowledge and skill of its leaders, and we ought not to judge the powers of medicine indiscriminately from the limitations of whoever may be licensed to practise. Notwithstanding this, the best of medicine is often powerless. I have already pointed out that however skilful diagnosis has become, it often makes mistakes. Disease is often a much more complex affair than its symptoms indicate, and scientific medicine has still much to learn regarding the interpretation of symptoms. When we pass from diagnosis to treatment, we find that "The best laid schemes o' mice and men gang aft agley." Drugs that stimulate do not always stimulate, and drugs that depress do not always depress. This remedy and that do not keep their promises. For a hundred times a course of treatment may succeed, and in the hundred and first time it fails. Unforeseen complications enter, and unknown conditions arise, and the patient steadily grows worse. Moreover, while medicine has achieved much, in every direction there are unsolved problems. The doctor can deal with diphtheria like magic, but he has no antitoxin for a cold in the head, or an attack of influenza. Rheumatism in his hands often thrives madly. He can skilfully remove or can stay the progress of a cancer, but a digestion that has given way after the accumulation of the gastric indiscretions of years he cannot cure in a day. A persistent high mortality from Bright's disease of the kidneys and various maladies of the heart reveals the growing need for their investigation.   When this occasional impotence of scientific medicine is disclosed in cases where one's own life or the lives of those near to one are at stake, it is perhaps not to be wondered at that, with emotions strongly aroused, one sometimes belittles the achievements that are already accomplished.

But if from tradition, his own ignorance, the inability of conventional medicine to do the impossible, or for any other reason, the individual has come to distrust the medical profession, what is he to do ?   Shall he seek relief in a medical sect, in homeopathy or eclecticism, or in such an aberrant school of healing as osteopathy ?   Or shall he fly to one of those several cults that offer a safe refuge to malcontents by promises of cure through psychic agencies ?   Shall he become a Christian Scientist, or a follower of one of the many other varieties of faith healing or of New Thought ?

It is interesting to watch the course of these protesting iconoclastic movements.   They present certain features in common.   Homeopathy with its elaborate dogma regarding drugs, its principle of "similia similibus curantur," its "potencies" and its "attenuations," arose in Germany a hundred years ago, but has gained its chief following in America.   It has already passed its zenith, and is now declining.   Its twenty-two medical schools existing in this country in 1900 had decreased to fifteen in 1910, and its student body had been diminished by one half.   The best of homeopathy has now assimilated itself to scientific medicine, and as a separate body it will undoubtedly soon cease to be.   Eclecticism represents a feeble survival of an effete medical system, and hardly deserves mention.

In osteopathy, on the other hand, we now have the oppor-

tunity to observe the rise of such a system. Osteopathy is
an outgrowth from the primitive conditions prevailing on our
western frontier in the period preceding our Civil War, when
educated physicians were few, opportunities for rational
treatment were fewer, and boldness in assertion and action
counted far more than exact conformity to scientific truth.
The founder of osteopathy was one of the rude, itinerant
practical bone-setters, probably often clever in his attitude
toward the sick. Though unlettered, he was possessed of a
positive philosophy that found a sympathetic hearing in the
home of many an unlearned frontiersman, who would have
been ill at ease under the ministrations of one trained in the
nice theories of academic medicine. Osteopathy was and still
is full of unfounded assertions regarding the normal func-
tioning of the bodily structures, and the nature and proper
methods of cure of disease, though of late years its more
enlightened practitioners appear to be endeavoring to harmonize its practices with certain accepted scientific principles. It speaks much of "lesions," by which it means, not
the commonly accepted pathological idea of morbid changes,
but rather "any structural perversion which by pressure
produces or maintains functional disorder." Of all parts of
the body subject to lesions the "spine" is of fundamental
importance, and "it is only in occasional cases of disease
that no treatment is given to it." Treatment consists chiefly
in correcting the structural perversion by manipulation with
the hands, and thus removing the pressure on the functionally disordered organs or on nerves and blood vessels supplying them. The osteopath serenely, with a single stroke of
the hand, waves away the facts of scientific pathology. Says
the prophet:

"I have concluded, after twenty-five years' close observation and experimenting, that there is no such disease as fever, flux, diphtheria, typhus, typhoid, lung-fever, or any other fever classed under the common head of fever. Rheumatism, sciatica, gout, colic, liver disease, nettle-rash, or croup, on to the end of the list of diseases, do not exist as diseases. All these, separate and combined, are only effects. The cause can be found, and does exist, in the limited and excited action of the nerves only, which control the fluids of parts or the whole of the body." The cause of all diseases is "a partial or complete failure of the nerves to properly conduct the fluids of life." One can with difficulty suppress a feeling of admiration for the audacity with which time-honored scientific facts and principles are thus put aside. Osteopathy undoubtedly effects cures, but so does the medicine man of the savage tribe.

Of the value and limitations of psychic agencies in the treatment of disease I have already spoken. It remains, however, to consider briefly some of those prominent sects in which mental healing overshadows all else. Christian Science, like osteopathy, had its rise in humble circumstances. In Phineas Parker Quimby, a clockmaker of New England, the germs of its philosophy seem to have originated; but in the visionary mind of Mary Baker Eddy they came to full fruition. Christian Science says that "Man is not matter, he is not made up of brain, blood, bones, and other material elements. . . . Man is idea. . . . Man is incapable of sin, sickness, and death." "Health is not a condition of matter, but of Mind." "What is termed disease does not exist." "If the body is diseased, this is but one of the beliefs of mortal mind." "We weep because others weep, we yawn because they yawn, and we have smallpox because others have it; but mortal mind, not matter, contains and carries the infection." "All disease is cured by divine Mind." "You say a boil is painful; but that is impossible, for matter without mind is not painful. The boil simply manifests, through inflammation and swelling, a belief in pain, and this belief is called a boil. Now administer mentally to your patient a high attenuation of truth, and it will soon cure the boil." "To reduce inflammation, dissolve a tumor, or cure organic disease, I have found divine Truth more potent than all lower remedies." "Decided types of acute disease are quite as ready to yield to Truth as the less distinct type and chronic form of disease. Truth handles the most malignant contagion with perfect assurance." "If the case to be mentally treated is consumption, take up the leading points included (according to belief) in this disease. Show that it is not inherited; that inflammation, tubercles, hæmorrhage, and decomposition are beliefs, images of mortal thought superimposed upon the body; that they are not the truth of man; that they should be treated as error and put out of thought. Then these ills will disappear." There is a certain type of mind that loves to play with thoughts like these. They require no depth of intellect or logic. They merely skim the surface of consciousness. It demands no great expenditure of mental power to learn the essentials of this crude metaphysics; and with that once mastered the whole field of medical possibility is before one.

When we read the records of the many cures that are claimed by Christian Science, we are impressed at first by the inexactness of the diagnoses. Thus we read of patients being cured of "a fever," "an internal disease," "an internal complaint," "liver complaint," and a long list of "troubles," such as "heart trouble," "stomach and bowel trouble," "abdominal trouble," "lung, liver, and kidney trouble," "neck trouble," "throat trouble," "nervous and spinal trouble." With such uncertainty as to the real nature of the diseases it is not strange that proof of cures is difficult to obtain. Among many others, Cabot, of Boston, has examined the evidence of a considerable number of such "cures." "In my own personal researches into Christian Science 'cures,'" he says, "I have never found one in which there was any good evidence that cancer, consumption, or any other organic disease had been arrested or banished. The diagnosis was usually either made by the patient himself or was an interpretation at second or third hand of what a doctor was supposed to have said. As I have followed up the reported cures of 'cancer' and other malignant tumors, I have found either that they were not tumors at all, or that they were assumed to be malignant without any microscopic examination. In other words, the diagnosis was never based upon any proper evidence. . . . By a curious process of 'natural selection,' a patient suffering from organic disease rarely consults a Christian Scientist, just as he rarely consults an osteopath. Being ignorant of diagnosis, the Christian Scientist is not aware of this fact, and supposes that he is treating, not a selected group of cases of functional disease, but all disease. This mistake is all the more natural, because the Christian Scientist, with the natural credulity of the half-educated, accepts the patient's own diagnosis at its face value or trusts the hearsay report of what some doctor is supposed to have said. . . . It is a striking fact that, as one listens to the recital of Christian Science 'cures,' one hears little or nothing of the great common organic diseases, such as arterio-sclerosis, phthisis, appendicitis — and still less of the common acute diseases, such as pneumonia, malaria, apoplexy. Chronic nervous (that is, mental) disease is the Christian Scientist's stock in trade."

Cabot's judgment does not differ essentially from that of others, and we must believe that as a therapeutic agent Christian Science is to be classed with the various other systems of mental healing, and is of very limited therapeutic application. Its ignorance of scientific medicine and its unwise extension into unwarranted fields are undoubtedly responsible for a vast amount of maltreatment of the sick and of unnecessary suffering. Its material success is due less to its merits as a system of healing than to other factors which appeal to the credulous, and it is undoubtedly destined to follow the course of its many vanished predecessors.

Supreme above all partisan healing sects and systems and creeds stands the scientific medicine of to-day, the heir of all that has preceded it since men began to heal. It asks itself these questions: What is health? What is disease? How may disease be prevented? How may the sick be cured? Its business is to discover and to apply the correct answers to these questions, and in doing this it exhibits the liberalism that characterizes all true science. It seeks its knowledge from all sources and by all legitimate means. All that it acquires it puts to the rigid, critical test of experiment, and it discards all that which does not stand this test. It thus represents a great body of selected scientific knowledge, which is the best that science can offer to-day. To-morrow its knowledge will be more abundant and more exact, and as science continually advances, medical science will keep pace. Its followers are terribly in earnest in their warfare against disease. Like the intrepid Ulysses, they are

> . . . " strong in will
> To strive, to seek, to find, and not to yield."

The altruism of men of medicine has become proverbial. Their heroism in investigating and treating disease is often put to the test, and is rarely found wanting. Their ideals are high, and they can be trusted to do what is within their power to put an end to the ills of suffering humanity. Yet it should be borne in mind that scientific medicine unaided has a well-nigh impossible work before it. If it is to accomplish the final banishment of disease, it must have the sympathetic coöperation and encouragement of mankind, in whose interests it continually labors.

INDEX

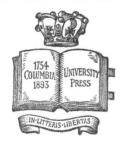

THE COLUMBIA UNIVERSITY PRESS

Columbia University in the City of New York

COLUMBIA UNIVERSITY LECTURES

BLUMENTHAL LECTURES

POLITICAL PROBLEMS OF AMERICAN DEVELOPMENT. By ALBERT SHAW, LL.D., Editor of the *Review of Reviews*. 12mo, cloth, pp. vii + 268. Price, $1.50 *net*.

CONSTITUTIONAL GOVERNMENT IN THE UNITED STATES. By WOODROW WILSON, LL.D., President of Princeton University. 12mo, cloth, pp. vii + 236. Price, $1.50 *net*.

THE PRINCIPLES OF POLITICS FROM THE VIEWPOINT OF THE AMERICAN CITIZEN. By JEREMIAH W. JENKS, LL.D., Professor of Political Economy and Politics in Cornell University. 12mo, cloth, pp. xviii + 187. Price, $1.50 *net*.

THE COST OF OUR NATIONAL GOVERNMENT. By HENRY JONES FORD, Professor of Politics in Princeton University. 12mo, cloth, pp. xv + 144. Price, $1.50 *net*.

THE BUSINESS OF CONGRESS. BY HON. SAMUEL W. McCALL, Member of Congress for Massachusetts. 12mo, cloth, pp. vii + 215. Price, $1.50 *net*.

JULIUS BEER LECTURES

SOCIAL EVOLUTION AND POLITICAL THEORY. BY LEONARD T. HOBHOUSE, Professor of Sociology in the University of London. 12mo, cloth, pp. ix + 218. Price, $150 *net*.

CARPENTIER LECTURES

THE NATURE AND SOURCES OF THE LAW. BY JOHN CHIPMAN GRAY, LL.D., Royall Professor of Law in Harvard University. 12mo, cloth, pp. xii + 332. Price, $1.50 *net*.

WORLD ORGANIZATION AS AFFECTED BY THE NATURE OF THE MODERN STATE. BY HON. DAVID JAYNE HILL, American Ambassador to Germany. 12mo, cloth, pp. ix + 214. Price, $1.50 *net*.

LEMCKE & BUECHNER, AGENTS
30–32 WEST 27th ST., NEW YORK

THE COLUMBIA UNIVERSITY PRESS

Columbia University in the City of New York

COLUMBIA UNIVERSITY LECTURES

HEWITT LECTURES

THE PROBLEM OF MONOPOLY. By JOHN BATES CLARK, LL.D., Professor of Political Economy, Columbia University. 12mo, cloth, pp. vi + 128. Price, $1.25 *net.*

POWER. By CHARLES EDWARD LUCKE, Ph.D., Professor of Mechanical Engineering, Columbia University. 12mo, cloth, pp. vii + 316. Illustrated. Price, $2.00 *net.*

THE DOCTRINE OF EVOLUTION. Its Basis and Scope. By HENRY EDWARD CRAMPTON, Ph.D., Professor of Zoölogy, Columbia University. 12mo, cloth, pp. ix + 311. Price, $1.50 *net.*

MEDIEVAL STORY AND THE BEGINNINGS OF THE SOCIAL IDEALS OF ENGLISH-SPEAKING PEOPLE. By WILLIAM WITHERLE LAWRENCE, Ph.D., Associate Professor of English, Columbia University. 12mo, cloth, pp. xiv + 236. Price, $1.50 *net.*

JESUP LECTURES

LIGHT. By RICHARD C. MACLAURIN, LL.D., Sc.D., President of the Massachusetts Institute of Technology. 12mo, cloth, pp. ix + 251. Portrait and figures. Price, $1.50 *net.*

SCIENTIFIC FEATURES OF MODERN MEDICINE. By FREDERIC S. LEE, Ph.D., Dalton Professor of Physiology, Columbia University. 12mo, cloth, vi + 183. Price, $1.50 *net.*

LECTURES ON SCIENCE, PHILOSOPHY, AND ART. A series of twenty-one lectures descriptive in non-technical language of the achievements in Science, Philosophy, and Art. 8vo, cloth. Price, $5.00 *net.*

LECTURES ON LITERATURE. A series of eighteen lectures on literary art and on the great literatures of the world, ancient and modern. 8vo, cloth, pp. 404. Price, $2.00 *net.*

LEMCKE & BUECHNER, AGENTS
30-32 WEST 27th ST., NEW YORK